The Ultimate Consumer Guide to Your Healthiest, Happiest Smile

by
Dr. Cary N. Goldberg
Dr. Charles J. Greenebaum

www.flossmoordental.com

Copyright ©2018 by Drs. Cary N. Goldberg and Charles J. Greenebaum.

All rights reserved. No part of this publication may be reproduced, distributed, or transmitted in any form or by any means, including photocopying, recording, or other electronic or mechanical methods, without the prior written permission of the publisher, except in the case of brief quotations embodied in critical reviews and certain other noncommercial uses permitted by copyright law.

Although the author and publisher have made every effort to ensure that the information in this book was correct at press time, the author and publisher do not assume and hereby disclaim any liability to any party for any loss, damage, or disruption caused by errors or omissions, whether such errors or omissions result from negligence, accident, or any other cause.

This book is not intended as a substitute for the medical advice of physicians. The reader should regularly consult a physician in matters relating to his/her health and particularly with respect to any symptoms that may require diagnosis or medical attention.

ISBN-13: 9781729257791

Dedication

To my father, Dr. Raymond Berlin ~

Your dedication to excellence in caring for your patients has been my example each and every day. And to my patients, who inspire me every day to provide the best service I can to make a positive difference in your lives.

– Dr. Cary Goldberg

To my father, Dr. Werner Greenebaum ~

A fine dentist who served as my role model in treating patients with compassion and empathy.

– Dr. Charles Greenebaum

Table of Contents

The Ultimate Consumer Guide i
    Dedication iii
    Foreword vi
What Makes our Office Unique x
What We Want Our Patients to Know xiii
    Why Is This Book So Important Today? xvi
Chapter 1 19
    Your Healthy Smile and Your Dentist: An Overview 19
    Life-Changing Stories 32
    Your Most Common Questions Answered 34
    Free Offer 36
Chapter 2 37
    Smile Makeovers 37
    Types of Smile Makeovers 43
    The Process of Your Smile Makeover 49
    Life-Changing Stories 51
    Your Most Common Questions Answered 53
    Free Offer 55
Chapter 3 57
    Dentures, Snap-In Dentures, Implants & All-On-4 57
    Your Options 66
    Life-Changing Stories 70
    Your Most Common Questions Answered 76
    Free Offer 80
Chapter 4 83
    Sleep Apnea Solved Without a CPAP Machine 83

Oral Appliance Therapy: Your Alternative to CPAP 88
Life-Changing Stories 89
Your Most Common Questions Answered.................................. 91
Free Offer 94

Chapter 5 95
Your Next Step 95
Your Free Offer 102

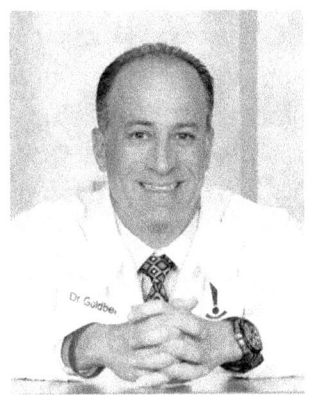

Cary N. Goldberg, D.D.S.

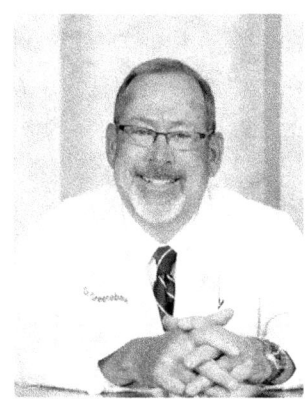

Charles J. Greenebaum, D.D.S.

Foreword

Let us introduce ourselves. We are Dr. Cary N. Goldberg and Dr. Charles J. Greenebaum. The first thing you should know about us is that we are a team; we have been a team since 1999 when we first merged our individual dental practices together to form a larger, more comprehensive practice. What started as two small, local dental practices evolved into a much larger, regional, nine-chair dental practice. Now, we are about to become a 20-chair, multi-specialty practice! What this expansion means is that we will have many dental specialties under one roof. If you need an implant placed by an Oral Surgeon, a root canal performed by an Endodontist, gum treatment by a Periodontist, braces by an Orthodontist or a Pediatric Dental specialist for your child, we will be able to provide all your care at our beautiful new state-of-the-art facility, rather than referring you elsewhere. In our existing practice, we already see patients of all ages, but soon our practice will truly be able to meet all the dental needs of any age patient. These needs range from maintaining optimal dental health to regular cleanings and examinations to cutting edge technology to improve smiles, improve the health of the teeth and gums and to treat all dental and orthodontic issues, no matter how simple or complex.

It has been an incredible journey and sometimes we have to pinch ourselves to verify that, yes, our childhood dreams have become reality in such an amazing way. It is almost like destiny that we have built our practice together because we grew up in such similar circumstances and had such similar childhood experiences. Our stories are so similar that they are basically versions of the same.

We come from a line of dentistry; both our Dads owned their own practices. We practically grew up in our Dads' offices and, in fact, both of us started working there by the time we were in Junior High School. It was great. We got to see how our Dads worked, and interacted, with their patients. We experienced how happy patients were when pain was taken away and smiles were restored. We watched our Dads solve problems and work hard to meet the needs of each and every one of their patients. We got to see how much the patients loved and respected our Dads, which was a wonderful thing to see as young kids. We learned at an early age that people don't think too much about their teeth until they have a problem; pain or a cavity or a cracked tooth, and then the problem becomes all-consuming because it is constant and, literally, in their faces. Our Dads were heroes to their patients in these situations. They could fix a broken tooth, take away pain or fill a cavity. We were intrigued by the creative and artistic aspects of dentistry. That's right; it wasn't all just about fixing teeth. It was skill, art and compassion all wrapped up in one.

We loved it and, honestly, we were both confident, early on, that we wanted to be just like our Dads. We had a strong desire to help people; to really make a difference in their everyday lives. We wanted to combine science, medicine and art and work creatively with our hands. So, we watched and learned and grew up, and here we are with an excellent practice of our own!

Dr. Goldberg went to dental school and obtained a Doctor of Dental Surgery degree from Northwestern University College of Dentistry in Chicago and Dr. Greenebaum received his Doctor of Dental Surgery from the University of Illinois College of Dentistry in Chicago. It was there that we combined our passions for wanting to make a real difference in peoples' lives and respect for our fathers' examples with a top-notch education. We learned the HOW of doing what we wanted to do and all the cutting-edge treatment and recommendations for being superior dental providers. We both graduated in the 1980's and went to work immediately as Doctors of Dental Surgery in our fathers' established practices.

It was 1999 when our amazingly parallel lives finally merged. Our fathers were retiring, and we wanted to find a partner to grow our individual dental practices. We found each other and decided to build our own new building and combine our efforts. We called our new practice, The Center for Dental Excellence and, since this merger; we have been striving to make sure that our practice is just that...*Excellent.*

Our Passion

We have a passion for making people happy. It is that simple. We love what we do and are very good at it. We want as many people as possible to benefit from this combination of our love for our work and our expertise in doing it. Dental pain is awful, and unsightly or diseased teeth can make people feel very ashamed and unhappy. As a result, they constantly hide their smile and learn to live with pain and embarrassment. This way of life is so unnecessary. There are many affordable options for repairing teeth and achieving a bright, beautiful, healthy smile.

We love the creativity offered us in making beautiful, healthy, well-functioning teeth. Form follows function. We always have aesthetics in mind as we improve the function of a patient's teeth, because we completely understand people's emotional desire for a beautiful smile, which is as important as their need for good function.

Often, patients come to us with a problem that causes pain and is embarrassing to them as well. If they look great and you made them comfortable during treatment, in addition to being out of pain when they leave, they're just incredibly happy, which makes us feel great. The gratitude, love and respect our patients have for us are some of the many reasons we're passionate about what we do.

Some of our most rewarding work is with patients who come to us in need of extensive restoration. We have seen many, many patients with very complex situations; people who are debilitated and handicapped because of their mouths; people who are truly unable to function. They can't eat the foods they want, and they don't feel good about themselves. Many of them have told us that they felt lost; like they couldn't see a way out of their situation. They have told us that they didn't know what to do or where to go; that they had seen other providers who didn't have the skill set or imagination to handle their issues. Or perhaps their issues were too complex, and their provider just didn't want to deal with them. These patients had lost hope and arrived at our office in desperation. We have restored the hope, health and confidence of so many patients in such challenging situations. You will meet a few of them in the pages that follow.

When I started practicing dentistry in 1982, if one of my patients needed a lower denture, they had basically reached bottom. There are lots of problems with an upper denture, but at least they tend to stay in place. A lower denture doesn't. It's very difficult. Now, do people learn how to function with them? Yes, they learn how, but it's not a very pleasant situation. So, in 1982, when a patient would come to me and say, "Hey Dr. Greenebaum, I have this denture down here, and I just can't wear it. Is there anything you can do to help me?" Besides making a new denture or relining the old one, there was little I could do. There was literally nothing that could truly improve their long-term situation.

Then, as technology developed, and implant dentistry became a reality, skilled dentists could replace teeth one at a time with dental implants. However, this one implant per tooth treatment was extremely costly and very time consuming. In addition, many patients weren't candidates for it or needed grafting or extensive surgery and a lot of time to devote to treatment in order to make it possible. In the late 1990's, a company called Nobel Biocare developed a treatment concept called, the All-on-4™. This amazing treatment technique, which we perform at The Center for Dental Excellence, allows patients in need of all new teeth to receive a set of new, beautiful, functioning teeth with just four implants. It has been designed in such a way that it is possible to perform the procedure on almost every person. It can even be done in just one day! Because it is so much easier, less expensive and less time consuming now, it is a restoration option available to many more people; not only the very wealthy. It has given tremendous hope to a very large population to know that they can eat again, smile again and enjoy their life again. The hope we see in our patient's eyes when we explain all these possibilities is exactly why we love what we do.

What Makes our Office Unique

We are unique in that we truly get to know our patients. We treat them with respect and never, ever judge them. We develop a relationship with each and every one of our patients and work very closely with each of them to develop a dental treatment plan. For example, we're not the kind of dental office where we come into the treatment room and say, "Okay, you need three fillings and two crowns. Go make an appointment at the front desk." No, we get to know our patients very well. We get to know not just what they need, but what they want; their specific situation and what is important to them. We talk about all the different alternatives and then we make a decision together about what the best treatment is for them in their own unique situation at this specific time in their lives. We are here to help them.

We are very much our patients' advocates; we're here to help them figure out the best plan for every situation. Whether they come to us in perfect dental health and just want a plan to maintain this health or they come to us with multiple problems that need significant work, we work tirelessly with them to ensure that their dental needs are met.

We also care deeply about the way people are greeted and treated in our office. We want every patient to be welcomed with a smile and to feel very comfortable; we don't want them to be scared and we certainly don't want them to experience pain. Indeed, our goal with every one of our patients is to help them forget that they are at the dentist's office. When patients schedule treatment at a dental office, it's not something they look forward to and many truly fear it. Our goal is to provide them with an experience they don't expect at a dental office - a fun atmosphere, with 5-star service, friendly, caring staff, individualized treatment and respect. We treat people the way we'd like to be treated. We respect their time. Our office culture and the quality of our dental treatment are what make us different and our patients talk about it all the time.

We are a dental office that specializes in flexibility. We know our patients' time is very limited, so our office hours are intended to meet their needs. We have extended weekday hours (before *and* after school or work) and Saturday hours. We also love providing same day dentistry. We know that dental pain or discomfort is awful, and we certainly do not want our patients to suffer. So, we make it a practice to provide same-day appointments for patients who need urgent help. However, this concept goes beyond having appointments available the same day. For example, if a patient comes in for a cleaning and a cavity is found, we'll take care of it that day instead of making the patient come back for a second appointment on yet another day. Our patients are busy, so we make the best use of their valuable time.

Another way we are unique is that we are able and willing to make treatment affordable. For example, we're able to perform treatments in phases over a period of time. We don't just tell the patient what they need and when they need it. We spend a lot of time with them and come up with a plan together. We think this approach is important and unique. We don't want our patients to worry about cost when they need dental care, so we are flexible when it comes to payments. We work with most dental insurance companies and take on the paperwork burden of obtaining cost estimates and filing insurance claims, so our patients don't have to. We also work with several companies to be able to offer 0% financing and we have low-interest options, which allow our patients to schedule treatments and pay on a monthly plan. For those patients not fortunate enough to have dental insurance, we offer an in-house dental savings plan for most services at an affordable yearly fee.

Our office is also unique in that we are all about giving forward to better our community. Since the founding of The Center for Dental Excellence, making a difference in our community has been at the heart of our practice. We love helping our community! In addition to providing state-of-the-art dental care, we support over forty non-profit organizations in our local community, including youth sports teams, local schools, community outreach programs and civic groups. We also love to support our patients in their charitable endeavors. One of our favorite days of the year is when we participate in Dentistry from the Heart. On this day, our practice is dedicated solely to meeting the dental needs of people in our community who do not have the financial means to afford dental care. Our team volunteers to provide all dental services on this day at zero cost to the patient. It is such an amazing experience to witness the happiness and gratitude of people who are finally able to have their teeth cleaned, a cavity filled or dental pain relieved. We are so grateful for the opportunity to use our skill and expertise to truly make a difference in the lives of people in our community. We see over 100 patients on this day and, at the end of the day, our whole staff is exhausted, but energized by this incredibly joyful experience. We love giving back to our local community as it has given so much to us.

What We Want Our Patients to Know

We're writing this book because we want to help people become more knowledgeable about dental care, including what to look for when choosing a quality dental practitioner, what experience to expect in a dental office, the cost of dental care and how to afford it.

We also really want our patients, potential patients and community members to be more prepared for common dental issues that affect themselves, their family and friends throughout the various stages of life. Even if people have great dental health and come in every 6 months for dental cleanings and examinations, problems can still occur. We want our patients to know that when problems do arise, we will be there for them and it won't be scary.

An example of the conversation that may come up if patients read our book may sound a lot like the following:

"You're in great health, and your teeth look really good. I just want you to know that you're probably going to have your teeth for a lifetime, but sometimes, things happen. You could even end up losing a tooth. We just want you to know that if a dental problem arises, we have the expertise to provide you with a variety of great solutions. We are able to do things today that weren't possible in the past. We will be here for you.

What's good about having this conversation early on is that if something does happen to a patient five years in the future and they lose a tooth, it's not the first time they've heard that this could be a possibility. It avoids the following thought patterns that a patient may have, "What the heck, I go there every six months; I'm not supposed to be losing a tooth!?"

Another reason we wrote this book is so that our current patients, potential patients and our community members know the range of treatments we provide. Some of our patients have actually gone to other offices to seek specific dental care because they were not aware that we offered it. That's on us.

We obviously didn't do a good job of informing these patients about all the services we perform. No more. We want to do a great job of communicating with our patients and this book is a great tool for sharing such information.

For us, it is all about community. We want the people in our community to know that we are the type of practice they would enjoy being part of. Perhaps they have had an unpleasant dental experience, or they just haven't been going to the dentist regularly. We want them to know that dentistry can be a very pleasant, even fun experience; that being in good dental health and having a nice smile will make their life better and better things will come to them as a result. We want people to know that they do not have to suffer; that there are always solutions to dental problems, even if they can't imagine what that solution might be.

We help break down the barrier that exists for the 50% of the adult population who don't go to the dentist on a regular basis. These people need to know that we are friendly, fun, pain free and affordable. They need to understand that regular dental visits are critical to preventing more serious health issues in the future. Dental problems left untreated only grow more complicated, more uncomfortable and more expensive. We are here to help keep all those unpleasantries at a minimum!

We also aim to be a calming presence for the potentially 60% of people who have fear and anxiety about going to the dentist and the 5%-10% of patients who have actual dental phobia. We even offer a Comfort Menu with a variety of relaxing items to choose from. We understand that fear or anxiety is very real, and we understand why. Many times, it comes from a series of bad childhood dental experiences or even from one very bad dental experience as an adult. We want to motivate people who are fearful of the dentist; to take that first step of visiting our office so they can see what we're like; that we're different and that their experience with us will be very different. We don't just brush off these feelings but help them relax and overcome their anxiety. It may not happen in one day, but it will happen. People need to see for themselves that not all dental offices are alike; that some, like ours, can actually make the experience of dental care a very positive one!

Our dental practice, The Center for Dental Excellence, received the South Suburban Small Business of the Year Award in 2017 in a region representing 79 different communities. We are honored by this distinction and so thankful to have a positive influence on this place we call home. Come see us and find out what an amazing experience it is to be a patient at The Center for Dental Excellence. We welcome the opportunity to be the dental solution for you, your friends, family, neighbors and coworkers:

Dr. Cary N. Goldberg, D.D.S
Dr. Charles J. Greenebaum, D.D.S

Why Is This Book So Important Today?

If you're reading this book, then chances are you may not be as happy with your smile as you would like to be. You might feel frustrated or self-conscious about your teeth. Maybe you're even living with pain in your mouth. Ultimately, we want to show that you don't have to suffer anymore. You can get back to living a normal life with a happy, healthy, and beautiful smile.

With the significant advances made in dental technology over the years and the modern materials that have been made available, now is an ideal time to see a dentist. Today, your trip to the dentist can result in a very realistic, long-lasting, and beautiful smile.

At *The Center for Dental Excellence,* we recognize that you have choices when it comes to your treatment. Our goal is to explain your different treatment options so that you can make the right decision for your unique needs. We are confident that you'll find the information we share to be beneficial.

As you read our book, you'll learn a great deal to help guide you when it comes to your smile. For example:

- You'll find 10 easy must-do steps for maintaining your healthy smile.

- You'll discover the top 10 keys to finding a dentist who is as dedicated to you as he or she is dedicated to your smile.

- We'll share some of the available smile makeover options for you to consider.

- You'll learn about some of the smile makeover

procedures we offer here at *The Center for Dental Excellence.*

- You'll learn how your initial consultation and examination with us can be 100% free. We will even include free x-rays to ensure that your diagnosis and analysis are fully accurate.

The bottom line is that, by the end of this book, you will know how to choose the right dentist for yourself *and* how to have a healthier and happier smile!

Chapter 1

Your Healthy Smile and Your Dentist: An Overview

10 Easy Must-Dos for Your Healthy Smile

1. Remember to brush and floss effectively every day.

Many of us learn from an early age that we're supposed to brush twice a day, but we don't always do it *effectively*. When you brush, make sure you're not rushing the process! Take at least two full minutes to brush your teeth. This lets your brushing regimen reach its full potential while you scrub away food particles and plaque.

For you to maintain your healthiest smile, it's also critical that you remember to floss at least once a day. Flossing removes stubborn food and plaque from between your teeth – the stuff your toothbrush can't reach – and helps to keep your gums happy.

Many other aids have been developed to help keep your teeth and gums healthy. The hygienists at CDE are always working to find the most effective solution for each individual patient's needs.

◇◇◇

2. Limit your intake of sweets.

You may already know that sugary foods can lead to tooth decay and cavities – but did you know why? According to the National Institute of Dental and Craniofacial Research (NIH), the sugar itself isn't what causes the decay, but rather the bacteria that live in our mouths.

You're not the only one with a sweet tooth; bacteria love sugar, too! When we avoid sugar, we starve out the bacteria and don't give them a chance to do any harm. When we *do* eat those sweets, though, we're enabling those bacteria to produce the acid that damages our tooth enamel.

3. Don't use tobacco.

In addition to yellowing your teeth, tobacco can damage your beautiful smile in several other ways. When you smoke, you're reducing your body's ability to fight off infection – including in your mouth. As a result, smokers have a higher risk of gum disease, mouth pain, and tooth loss.

Don't think you're out of the woods if you use an alternative to cigarettes such as snuff, chewing tobacco, or cigars, either! In addition to increasing your risk of cancer in your cheeks or gums, these alternative forms of tobacco also introduce abrasive particles into your mouth that can wear down your teeth over time.

4. Use a mouth guard when you play sports.

Few things can ruin the enjoyment of playing a sport as much as a sudden impact to the mouth. From a lacerated lip to a chipped or dislocated tooth, the resulting injury can end up being painful and expensive to fix. By wearing a mouth guard, you can minimize the risk to your healthy smile.

You can buy a "boil-and-bite" mouth guard at the store, or you can talk to your dentist for a custom-fit mouth guard. Both work the same way: they redistribute the force of the impact to your mouth and thus limit the risk of damage.

5. Find a quality dentist who makes you feel comfortable and who values good communication.

Having an open channel of communication with your dentist not only decreases your anxiety during your visits; it also helps to ensure that you fully understand all your treatment options before beginning any new procedure. At *The Center for Dental*

Excellence, for example, you will find that open communication and patient comfort are two of our top priorities.

6. Keep up professional maintenance with regular trips to your dentist.

Even if you are a model example of at-home mouth care – avoiding sweets and remembering to brush and floss – you still need regular visits to your dentist. At these visits, your dentist will remove the resistant plaque and tartar that regular brushing can't get off your teeth. If not removed by your dentist, tartar can build up over time and lead to a number of oral diseases. A regular preventative visit will also give your dentist the chance to identify any cavities or other issues while they are still in their early stages and easier to correct.

7. Protect against tooth decay by using fluoride and sealants.

Your use of a fluoride-based toothpaste will play a huge role in keeping cavities at bay. In addition, while fluoride helps to strengthen the smooth surfaces of your teeth, sealants will address those tricky crevices that brushing and flossing can't reach. Your dentist applies sealants onto the chewing surface of your molars, and this preventive coating keeps food particles and plaque from damaging your tooth. In this way, sealants provide a great way to avoid unnecessary and costly cavities.

8. Whiten your teeth optimally with a quality dentist rather than with over-the-counter products.

Over-the-counter products such as tooth-whitening agents can be far less effective than treatments provided by your dentist – not to mention risky! When you see your dentist from the start, you know you won't end up needing expensive professional care to undo any damage caused by over-the-counter products.

9. Protect yourself from harmful habits such as tooth grinding.

If you wake up in the morning with a mild headache or a sore jaw, you might be grinding your teeth in your sleep. Repetitive tooth grinding can cause major problems over time, including tooth loss and jaw injury. Happily, there are ways to address tooth grinding, such as using a special mouth guard at night. You can talk to us here at *The Center for Dental Excellence* if you'd like to learn how to protect yourself from the destructive effects of grinding and clenching.

◇◇◇

10. Don't wait if you notice signs of dental disease. Get treatment right away!

If you're experiencing mouth pain, have bleeding gums or concerns about your teeth, don't wait to visit your dentist! The longer you put off addressing a problem, the more difficult and expensive it will be to fix later. By treating dental disease as soon as it occurs, you will safeguard your healthy smile for years to come.

10 Keys to Choosing Your Dentist

#1: Does your dentist offer same-day emergency appointments?

Let's face it. When your tooth hurts, it can hurt just as much to hear that your dentist can't offer you an appointment for several days, if not weeks. Be sure to find out whether your potential new dental team will be available if you are in pain or have an emergency. You may often find that dental practices are booked weeks in advance, leaving little wiggle room for emergency visits. You should feel confident that when you need your dentist, the whole team will be there for you.

For example, at *The Center for Dental Excellence,* you are always our number one priority. We know what tooth pain feels like and how important it is to bring you relief. We keep openings in our schedule to cater to our patients, both new and existing, for when they are feeling pain. If you call us in the morning, we will be able to see you that afternoon. If you call in the afternoon, we will figure out a way to help you as soon as possible.

◇◇◇

#2: Does your dentist offer same-day treatment?

Whether you are visiting your dentist as a new patient or for a routine checkup, the last thing you want to hear is that you need to come back for a second appointment before your treatment can actually begin. After the dentist identifies any potential issue and decides the course of treatment, it can be days or even weeks later before the actual treatment begins. Unfortunately, this is how many dental offices set up their schedules.

To avoid the hassle and potential ongoing discomfort that this process can cause, ask your potential dental office whether they offer same-day starts for treatment. In other words, ask them if your initial appointment includes enough time not only for your exam and consultation, but also for your actual treatment if you decide to proceed.

At *The Center for Dental Excellence*, we value your time and busy schedule. That's why we give our patients the option, whenever possible, to have their treatment taken care of on the same day.

◇◇◇

#3: Does your dentist offer flexible scheduling?

Many dental offices have office hours that only span the hours of a regular workday, Monday through Friday. Some aren't even open on Fridays or Wednesdays – never mind the weekends! This means you'll likely have to leave work or school just for a routine appointment, causing you to miss important curriculum or paid wages. In addition, some dentists' schedules can be tightly pre- scheduled for months, leaving few options to line up with your own schedule.

At *The Center for Dental Excellence,* we want to work with your schedule. We know that it's difficult to spare the time for a routine appointment while you're working or at school. That is why we have adapted our hours to include appointment availability both before and after your typical work and school day. Additionally, we have Saturday hours to accommodate even the most rigid of schedules. If you find that our current hours still don't work for your schedule, let us know! We will do the best we can to accommodate you.

◇◇◇

#4: Can your dentist provide a similar case with results?

When you arrive for your appointment to address tooth pain, your dentist may explain that you have "irreversibly inflamed pulp tissue in your lower right first bicuspid" and that he'll need to perform a root canal to salvage the tooth. But what does that mean? Are you being upsold? Is there another solution? Can your dentist explain it to you in simple terms? Can he show you a similar case, note the similarities, and provide images of successful results? If not, you should seek a second opinion before committing to any procedure.

Improper diagnosis and incorrectly applied dental procedures can lead to more problems and more pain further down the line. At *The Center for Dental Excellence,* no matter what your dental situation may be, we have likely encountered and resolved a similar case that we can share with you.

◇◇◇

#5: Does your dentist offer any satisfaction guarantees?

Most dental offices aren't willing to stand behind their treatments to ensure your satisfaction. *The Center for Dental Excellence* is glad to offer you a 100% satisfaction guarantee on work provided.

◇◇◇

#6: Is your dentist nationally recognized?

Many dentists complete their schooling, serve their residencies, and assume proficiency in their field. Once fully certified in the field of dentistry, they no longer strive to achieve regional or national recognition. They simply rely on their certification for their credibility.

Our dentists and *The Center for Dental Excellence* have received both regional and national recognition. We feel it's important for our current and future patients to know that we not only meet the rigid standards of dental associations, but also exceed them.

Our dedication to high-quality dentistry has been recognized multiple times, too. *The Center for Dental Excellence* was honored to receive the South Suburban Small Business of the Year Award, representing 79 local communities. We were also voted the Patch Reader's Choice Award for Best Dental Office and have earned the Angie's List Super Service Award for multiple years running. We have 5-star reviews on Facebook, Healthgrades, Yelp, and Google. In addition, we are accredited by the Better Business Bureau with an A+ rating. We are proud of our many accomplishments and accreditations, as they symbolize what our patients and community overwhelmingly think of us! Being nationally recognized exemplifies that we constantly strive to improve our standards for providing exceptional care.

◇◇◇

#7: Does your dentist give back to the community?

There is a lot that can be said about a dental practice that not only has a presence in their community, but also strives to nurture growth and development. Some practices are glad to donate to one or two causes – but is that enough of a contribution?

At *The Center for Dental Excellence,* we believe it is essential to support local organizations in order to better the community in which we live and work. We also donate our time and service by providing free dental care to Veterans and through an international program called *Dentistry from the Heart.*

Ultimately, we find that our presence in the community reaffirms the way that we treat our patients like family.

◇◇◇

#8: Does your dentist have a comfortable environment?

It's no secret that many people feel anxiety about their dental visits, but that doesn't necessarily have to be the case! Seek out a dental team who appreciates the importance of comfort. You should ensure that the office is sterile and clean while still maintaining a warm and friendly atmosphere to help you feel at home.

At *The Center for Dental Excellence,* we recognize how essential it is to provide an extremely clean, comfortable environment for you – but we like to take it a step even further by offering your own unique Comfort Menu. This menu is all about you!

Here are some examples of the items you can request during every visit:

- Coffee, tea, cider and water
- Neck support pillow
- Personal earbuds
- Stress reliever
- Sunglasses
- Free WiFi
- Warm blankets
- Lip Balm

We give you this Comfort Menu to make your experience more enjoyable and calming. It really is all about you when you visit us here at *The Center for Dental Excellence.*

Take, for example, one of our general dental patients who decided to have a smile makeover done. She took the time to describe her experience with us:

"Not one time was the treatment uncomfortable. No tooth ache, not even after gum surgery. It was all SO worth it. I feel younger. I now have a big smile, and my teeth really show. People still compliment me all the time as they notice my beautiful teeth. Even strangers! I really appreciate the fact that I can get a response from *The Center for Dental Excellence* at any time. I will never forget that Dr. Goldberg opened the office just to see me on a summer Saturday when I had a dental emergency. They always make you feel so comfortable."

∞∞

#9: Does your dentist have the latest technology?

Many dental offices do not regularly upgrade their technology. Some don't even use digital x-rays yet! When an office doesn't have the latest, most innovative, and most effective technology available, this can lead to additional office visits, which then increases your treatment costs. Additionally, not utilizing the latest technology can lead to inferior treatment.

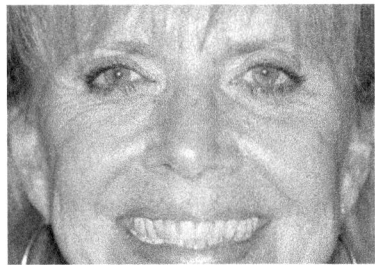

At *The Center for Dental Excellence*, we are constantly updating our technology to provide the highest possible standard of dental care.

For example, look at the **three photos to the left**. Notice both the discoloration of the teeth and their inconsistent appearance in the top "before" picture. You might assume that the middle picture here is her "after" photo, but that is actually a computer-generated image of her projected "after treatment" photo!

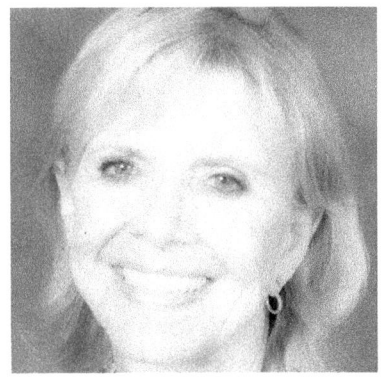

The patient's *real* "after" picture is **on the bottom**. Notice how close the computer-generated image is to the actual "after" photo. This type of technology allows you to see what your smile will look like before any procedure even begins.

This is just a sample of the state-of-the-art technology we use at *The Center for Dental Excellence*, so we can offer you the best possible dental care.

#10: Does your dentist have a full-service dental office?

Many dental offices aren't equipped to provide more than dental cleanings and basic dental work, such as cavity fillings. If you want any cosmetic procedures, or if you need help with your gums or other dental problems, this more traditional type of dental office may need to send you somewhere else.

At *The Center for Dental Excellence,* we're a full-service dental practice. Do you need a comprehensive dental exam and cleaning? Are you interested in a complete smile makeover or dentures? Do you need help with gum recession, or do you even want to permanently replace all your teeth? We can help you with it all! Our doctors are highly trained and have years of experience providing the highest level of care. You'll also find that our entire staff at *The Center for Dental Excellence* will treat you with the utmost respect. In fact, we hear from patients every day who say they love coming to our warm, friendly office.

◇◇◇

Since we always love to "over deliver" at The Center for Dental Excellence, we decided to include one more key item that you must know before choosing your dentist:

#11: Does your dentist offer flexible payment options?

Most dental offices accept insurance, but some require you to file the paperwork on your own. Most dentists also take credit cards and offer financing options for procedures – but that is typically the extent of their customer service support.

At *The Center for Dental Excellence,* we don't think anyone should go without high-quality dental care for any reason, especially financial ones. We process almost all insurance plans, and we will gladly work with your insurance company to ensure you receive the maximum benefit. We also offer 0% financing and flexible payment terms to help meet your budget. We take all major credit cards, *and* we also have an in-house savings plan for those of you who don't have dental insurance.

Because we care about you and your dental health, we've created the Dental Assistance Savings Plan to make our dental services more attainable and affordable. In exchange for a small annual membership fee, you receive your preventive dental care at no charge, and you also gain access to great discounts on many other dental procedures. This program includes:

- At least 2 preventative cleanings per year for $0
- X-Rays for $0
- Exam for $0
- Fluoride for $0
- There are NO claim forms
- There are NO exclusions
- There is NO waiting period
- There are NO yearly maximums
- And there are NO deductibles

This is just one of the many ways we make dental treatment affordable for you here at *The Center for Dental Excellence.*

Life-Changing Stories

Pictured here is one our patients who had all her lower and upper teeth replaced in only one day. After her procedure, she told us, "I feel younger. I feel great about myself, as my self-confidence has improved. I feel that this experience has given me a second chance to be that person I have always wanted to be. I have a new set of teeth, and no one knows the difference."

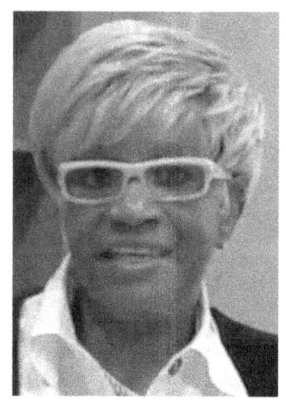

In fact, this patient felt so wonderful about her new teeth that it affected her overall health. She even lost 13 pounds after the procedure! Overall, between shedding some weight and gaining her new smile, she said "I really feel great about myself."

Now we can't promise that you will lose weight because of our implants. Just like with many of our patients, though, you may very well find that a healthier mouth can lead to a healthier life.

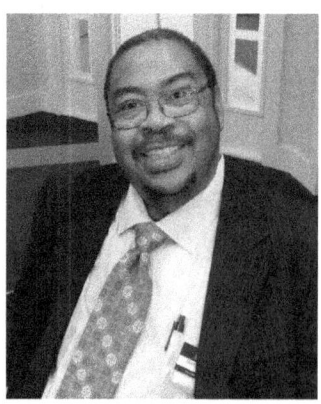

Another patient of ours, pictured here on the left, had us make him dentures. He'd had horrible experiences at several other offices, despite their good reputations. He had spent a fortune – several thousand dollars – and experienced lots of pain, yet he still had no resolution. His teeth were deteriorating.

He arrived apprehensively to meet with us at *The Center for Dental Excellence.* His upper teeth were beyond salvation, so we made him an upper plate. It fit his mouth comfortably and snugly. Then we went to work on his lower teeth to prevent any further deterioration. He has since reported that he has no pain or sensitivity issues anymore. "I am amazingly satisfied," he told us. "My whole attitude has improved. Dr. Greenebaum's treatment gave me the ability to smile again. Dr. Greenebaum is one of the few people who I have no inhibition in recommending to others."

You may be surprised to learn how little time it took for these amazing transformations to be completed. After her initial consultation and exam, the first patient with All-on-4 had her new smile after spending just one morning in our office, and the second patient with dentures only needed a few visits. In both cases, the end results were phenomenal and changed their lives.

Whether you need to see one of our hygienists for preventive care or want advice from one of our dentists about the current state of your teeth, we are here to help you. In every circumstance, our number-one goal is to maximize your safety while we minimize your discomfort.

Your Most Common Questions Answered

QUESTION: I've never been to the dentist. Will you still see me at *The Center for Dental Excellence*?

ANSWER: Of course! We will make your visit enjoyable and help ensure that your mouth is healthy.

QUESTION: Are these dental procedures painful?

ANSWER: That is a very common question. There is no discomfort associated with most procedures. In fact, even with complex treatment like the "All on 4" procedure (where we remove all remaining teeth and replace them with permanent teeth), those patients told us even *that* procedure wasn't painful. Any mild discomfort is generally controlled with over-the-counter Tylenol or Advil.

QUESTION: Another dentist told me I don't have enough bone for implants. Should I still come and see you?

ANSWER: Absolutely! You probably *do* have enough bone. We will use a state-of-the art CT scan to confirm your diagnosis. We urge you to contact us and make an appointment. We look forward to talking with you!

QUESTION: I currently don't have insurance. How do I get your Dental Assistance Savings Plan?

ANSWER: The application is a simple form you fill out. We will go over that in greater detail during your first visit, and we can typically get same-day approvals.

QUESTION: Is there a fee for using your computer-generated smile technology at *The Center for Dental Excellence*?

ANSWER: As part of your initial consultation for your smile makeover, there is no fee for using our imaging technology. We want you to see how great your results will look after treatment!

Free Offer

To schedule your consultation, head over to our website at www.YourFreeDentalConsult.com or simply call us at (708) 866-0063.

There is no obligation and this consultation is 100% free.

We want you to feel better, look better and ultimately live better. Patients tell us all the time that coming to see us is a life-changing experience for them. They tell us they can once again talk, laugh, and eat comfortably with family, friends, and co-workers. They no longer feel hostage to their teeth.

We want you to have that same transformation, so contact us now to schedule your free consultation. We look forward to seeing you very soon!

Chapter 2

Smile Makeovers

Overview

Imagine what your life would be like if you never had to worry about hiding your teeth – if you could stop feeling embarrassed about your smile. Visualize how it would feel if you had that smile you always wanted and had the ability to eat anything without trouble.

What would that feel like? Pretty amazing, right?

Now consider another question. How will your life be if you don't learn more about these different procedures that can change your life? What will life be like if you don't smile because you're embarrassed about your teeth? How will this affect you physically, emotionally, and even socially?

In this chapter, we're going to show you a variety of methods that can provide you with a complete set of fully functional and beautiful teeth. You can enjoy smiling again, improve your confidence, eat all the foods you want without a challenge, and even have an overall healthier lifestyle.

We are so excited to tell you how your ultimate smile transformation can become a reality!

We simply love helping our patients achieve the smiles they've always dreamt about. You'll be amazed to see that many, *many* of our transformations are simple modifications that can make such a huge difference to your smile and overall life. Oftentimes, you don't have to change every tooth completely to make a significant difference. The phrase "Smile Makeover" may sound like a lot of work, but in reality, a smile makeover doesn't always need to be extensive.

Here is what you'll learn in this chapter:

- The myths and misconceptions around smile makeovers;
- Information about many of the smile makeover procedures that we perform at *The Center for Dental Excellence;*
- How the smile makeover process works;
- How a smile makeover at any age will help you gain confidence and feel great.

In summary, by the end of this chapter you will know more about the types of techniques available for your own smile makeover – techniques that can help you acquire more confidence and enjoy a better life.

6 Misconceptions about Smile Makeovers

Misconception #1: Age is a factor when considering a smile makeover.

Age is *definitely* not a factor.

We can perform smile makeovers on young people, older people, and everyone in between. People of all ages color their hair, get new glasses, use the latest cosmetics, wear nice clothes, and take pride in their appearance. In fact, we often hear patients wish that they hadn't waited as long as they did to get their smile makeover. The sooner you get the procedure done, the more years you can have to enjoy life fully.

◇◇◇

Misconception #2: Smile makeover procedures are painful.

Typically, there is no discomfort during or after the procedure. During the procedure itself, you're in a pleasant environment, and we closely monitor your comfort level at all times. Afterward, any mild soreness can be alleviated with over-the-counter Tylenol or Advil. Some procedures do not even require any anesthetic!

◇◇◇

Misconception #3: You think you are not a candidate for a smile makeover.

Everyone is a candidate for a smile makeover – whether you have all of your teeth, some of your teeth, or none of your teeth.

Misconception #4: Teeth whitening is expensive.

In fact, teeth whitening is quite affordable, and you'll get more value from a professional whitening treatment than from the weaker at-home kits you can buy at the store.

There's a big difference between the results of a teeth whitening procedure performed in a dental office and the results from an over-the-counter kit. Because we supervise the procedure, a stronger bleaching solution can be used than that found in home kits. Additionally, our office has ZOOM! in-office whitening is equipped to use a light or heat source, so you can achieve stunning same-day results.

◇◇◇

Misconception #5: Smile makeovers require major procedures.

The reality is, a chipped tooth can sometimes be fixed in under 30 minutes. Having a smile that you're proud of doesn't necessarily require major procedures.

◇◇◇

Misconception #6: Smile makeovers are unaffordable.

That couldn't be further from the truth. *The Center for Dental Excellence* offers procedures that fit into almost any budget. We also process most dental insurances and will advocate for you to maximize your benefits.

If you don't have dental insurance, we offer an in-house dental assistance savings plan to save you money and make your treatment more affordable. Some of our patients have also used their Health Savings Accounts or Flex Spending Accounts for their smile makeovers.

Additionally, we have 0% financing plans available and we accept all major credit cards. We have many affordability options that will fit your budget. There may even be tax benefits for you. The truth is, everyone's circumstance is different – so the cost of your smile makeover will vary. The best way to get an accurate idea of what yours will cost is to come in for your free consultation with us.

Types of Smile Makeovers

Bonding

Tooth bonding is used for a variety of purposes:
- Close tooth gaps
- Cover discolorations
- Repair chipped or cracked teeth

Tooth bonding is dependent on the artistic ability of the dentist since the work is done "freehand" and no laboratory is used. The tooth must be color matched, sculpted, and polished to produce a beautiful and natural-looking result.

All our dentists at *The Center for Dental Excellence* are specially trained in tooth bonding techniques and have many years of experience in cosmetic dentistry – not to mention a natural flair for creating beautiful teeth!

Bonding procedures are typically performed in just one visit. Sometimes, however, several procedures are indicated. In the picture below, for example, the patient received Invisalign treatment to straighten his teeth before we filled the gaps with bonding. The end result? A happy patient with a handsome, confident smile!

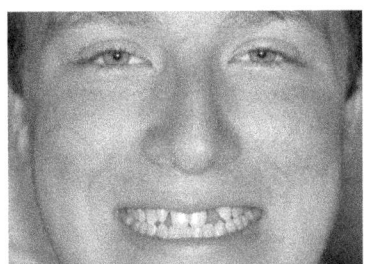
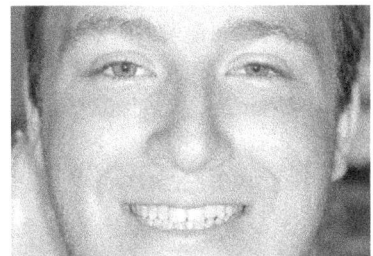

Dental Crowns

We often recommend placing a crown when a tooth is cracked, has an old filling, or is severely decayed. A crown covers a damaged tooth to strengthen and protect the remaining tooth structure. Crowns can also improve your smile by restoring the appearance of damaged teeth.

Porcelain Veneers

A porcelain veneer is just that: a thin layer of porcelain bonded to the tooth's surface. Veneers are a more conservative alternative for improving your smile's appearance.

Veneers can be used to:

- Close spaces between the teeth
- Fix broken or chipped teeth
- Whiten permanently stained or discolored teeth
- Fix crooked or misshapen teeth

Veneers are often referred to as "instant orthodontics," because they can provide an aesthetic transformation with minimal tooth preparation. In fact, your beautiful smile makeover using veneers can be completed in as little as two visits.

Tooth-Colored Restorations

Tooth-colored restorations are made of tooth-colored resin or porcelain. When filling a cavity, they create a more natural-looking smile than silver fillings do.

Tooth-colored restorations can also be used to:

- Restore teeth that are cracked or fractured if the damage is not severe enough to require a crown;

- Replace outdated and unattractive gray-silver fillings;
- Replace old yellow fillings in the front of your mouth;
- Cover dark, exposed roots.

Overall, their use helps to conserve much of your tooth's natural structure.

Invisalign

Invisalign has changed the face of orthodontics. Instead of wires attached to your teeth, your teeth can now be straightened invisibly. You can straighten your teeth *without anyone knowing!*

Unlike with braces, you can eat and drink whatever you want during Invisalign treatment. You can also brush and floss normally to maintain good oral hygiene. With Invisalign, there aren't any metal brackets or wires to cause mouth irritation, and you'll experience less time in the dentist's chair getting adjustments.

Using Invisalign is actually a very simple process. The aligners are made through a combination of your dentist's expertise and 3-D computer-imaging technology. Invisalign can help correct a variety of problems with your teeth, including crowded teeth, widely spaced teeth, a crossbite, an overbite, or an underbite.

The Center for Dental Excellence is a certified Invisalign provider.

Teeth Whitening

Teeth whitening is a procedure that removes stains and discoloration from your teeth. Discoloration can be the result of a combination of things:

- Genetics
- Poor oral hygiene

- Accidents
- Medication
- Effects of aging
- Smoking
- Certain foods or beverages

The whitening process is quick, easy, and comfortable. Under our dentist's supervision, your whitening treatment is completely safe and will not harm your teeth or gums.

At our office, we use the *ZOOM!* in-office whitening system because it's safe, effective, and very fast. The process is also simple! With proper care and an occasional touch-up at home, your brightened smile will sparkle for years. With in-office whitening, your teeth will be dramatically whiter after only 90 minutes. *Zoom!* whitening is ideal for anyone looking for immediate results. The convenience of *Zoom!* – in comparison to days of wearing trays for gradual whitening – makes it the perfect choice for the busy patient. Nothing whitens better or faster.

We also offer in-home whitening kits under our supervision. These whitening treatments are completely safe and will not harm your teeth or gums. With a professionally supervised at-home kit, you place a whitening gel into the custom trays at home and wear it for approximately 2-4 hours each day for a 2 to 4-week period.

The advantage of using dentist-supervised bleaching is that your teeth can be properly assessed to receive the precise chemical concentration, correct method, and proper length of treatment. We also make sure that you are an appropriate candidate for teeth whitening.

Gum Reshaping

A beautiful smile shows most of the 8 to 10 upper teeth with almost no gum above the two front teeth. If a significant amount of the gums can be seen in someone's smile, then their smile is considered "gummy."

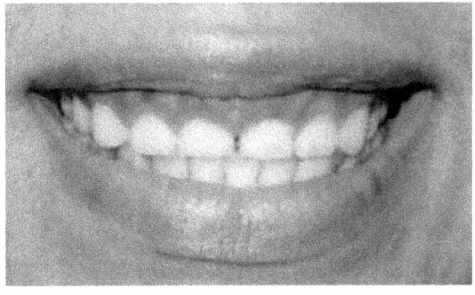

Although a gummy smile is considered a normal variation of human anatomy, many people with gummy smiles feel self-conscious about their appearance. Fortunately, these smiles can be corrected with a simple, minimally-invasive procedure. We safely modify the position and shape of your gums so that more of your natural enamel and less gum shows when you smile. You can see a before-and-after pictured here where the gums were reconstructed.

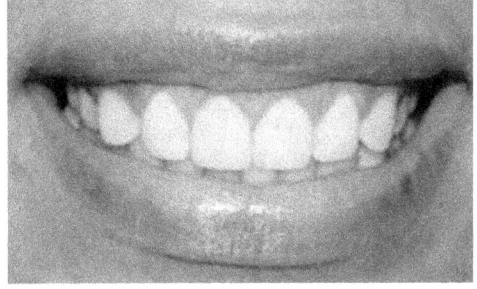

Sometimes, the opposite may happen, where you have the long-in-the-tooth look such as you see in the bottom left picture. Often, this type of issue is the result of gum recession. In addition to affecting the appearance of your smile, gum recession can also make your teeth sensitive to hot or cold foods and liquids.

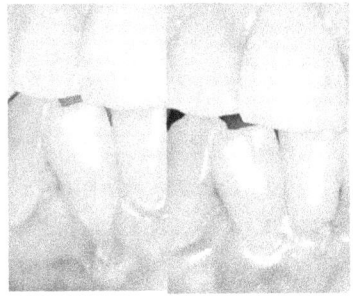

The solution to this problem is to cover one or more of the roots that make your teeth appear too long. We do this with a procedure called gum grafting, which can be done on one tooth or multiple teeth. Gum grafting can even your gum line and reduce sensitivity, as shown in the picture on the right.

Facelift Dentures

Did you know that dentures can be used to help give you a facelift? If you have a denture that was made years ago, we can now improve the look not only of your teeth, but of your face as well. We can reduce wrinkles, improve your profile, and ultimately give you a more natural, youthful look.

All-On-4

An All-on-4 procedure places four titanium implants in such a way that the bone will envelop and secure them into place. The implants that are placed in the back part of the jaw are angulated to achieve maximum advantage to the existing bone.

When you decide to move forward with the treatment, we can place your implants and fit your new replacement teeth all in the same day. Because only four implants are used in the procedure, the entire process is far less complicated and more affordable than older treatment options.

Remember, your teeth will be permanent and fixed, so there won't be any need for you to be without teeth or to endure temporary removable dentures for an extended time period. You can come in for a morning appointment and leave that same afternoon with a brand new, radiant smile!

Botox & Dermal Fillers

Now you may be wondering: what is the advantage of having Botox done at a dental office? There are three reasons. First, our dentists at *The Center for Dental Excellence* administer shots very gently. Second, we know facial anatomy extremely well. Third, Botox and fillers work seamlessly together with cosmetic dentistry to enhance your smile. Indeed, a dentist offering Botox and dermal fillers can be a perfect match for your needs.

The Process of Your Smile Makeover

The process for a smile makeover will vary from patient to patient. Initially, you will need a consultation and diagnostic appointment. This could include taking x-rays, making molds of your teeth, taking photographs of your teeth, and running computer simulations to preview what your smile could look like. Once we have done that, we can then determine your unique treatment path.

What Is Computer Simulation?

Take a look at these pictures:

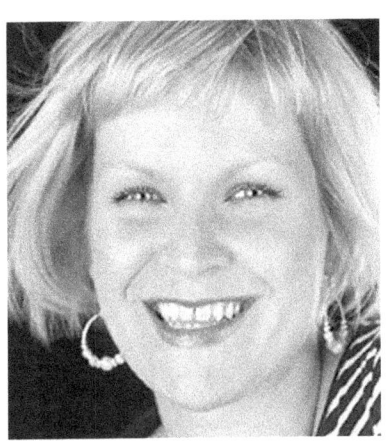 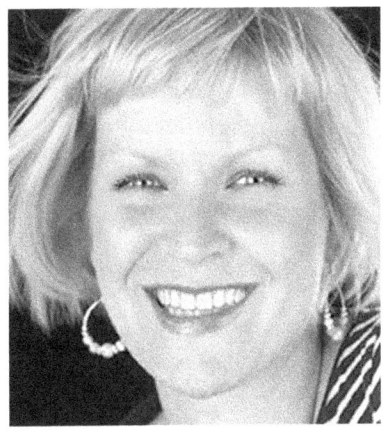

On the left, you can see the "before" photo with gaps, crooked teeth, and discoloration. You might think the picture on the right is her "after" photo, but it is actually a computer-generated image produced here at *The Center for Dental Excellence!*

Ultimately, you have two options.

Option #1: You could do nothing. With this option, you will probably continue to hide your smile. If you're in pain, your pain will most likely get worse. Let's face it, the option of doing nothing doesn't really make sense. You do not have to live with pain or hide your smile any longer.

Option #2: Take some time to speak with a dentist at *The Center for Dental Excellence*. We are all highly trained in every procedure reviewed in this book. Your consultation is 100% free, and you are under no obligation. We would love the chance to talk more about your specific mouth and your needs. We can discuss your options, and together we can customize a plan for your unique needs and desires. This option provides a wonderful, easy way for you to get your questions answered and understand your potential treatment paths.

Life-Changing Stories

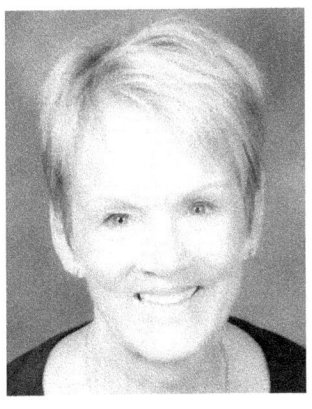

This patient lived with problematic soft teeth and had multiple bad dental experiences as a child. She lost some teeth in the back of her mouth and ended up with a nuisance of a bridge that eventually failed altogether.

As she was debating the qualifications of three potential new dentists, Dr. Goldberg gave her a call to see how she was doing and to find out if she had any additional questions that he could answer. That call helped her feel comfortable, so she decided to come in and talk more with him.

The connection and chemistry with her doctor was a very important factor in her decision. She felt that strong connection not only with Dr. Goldberg, but with every team member she encountered here at *The Center for Dental Excellence.* At our office, we have a fine-tuned process and a unique culture. Our team expresses genuine care and concern for our patients because we genuinely *do* care.

After her experience with us, this patient asserted, "I have never received this level of care at another office. There is something magical here." She said the friendship and camaraderie, coupled with the excellent care she was receiving, made her look forward to every dental visit. She couldn't wait to have her next treatment completed.

"I feel good about myself and comfortable in my own skin," she told us after her smile makeover. "My self-esteem has improved. I love that it's a permanent solution and wished I could have skipped the temporary fixes from other dentists that failed and had to be redone by Dr. Goldberg. It's the best investment I've made in myself. My husband thinks we should advertise 'Designer Smiles by Dr. Goldberg.'"

To other patients considering treatment, she says don't hesitate or delay. Hers was a fairly involved case, but the end result was amazing and changed her life.

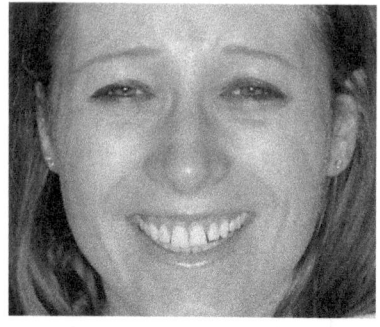

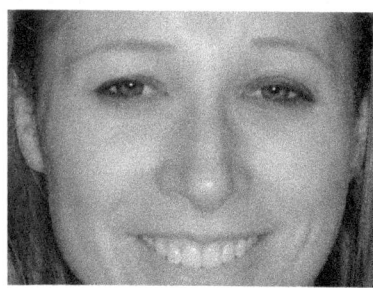

Now let's consider a far less involved case. For this patient on the left, we did some simple bonding to her teeth. We didn't take impressions or need a laboratory. Look at the "before" photograph on the top compared to her "after." This procedure was done in less than 60 minutes and in a single visit!

Our point in showing you these two extreme examples is that *The Center for Dental Excellence* can help you with all types of modifications to your mouth, from major to minor. In all circumstances, we comfortably create amazing smile makeovers.

Your Most Common Questions Answered

QUESTION: I have an important event coming up in just a couple weeks, and I would love a smile makeover. Are there procedures that can be done within this time frame? Are you available?

ANSWER: We certainly have procedures that can be done in a relatively short time frame, and we do have consultation appointments available on short notice. In fact, we can even typically schedule your consultation for the same day that you call us.

◇◇◇

QUESTION: Are these procedures painful?

ANSWER: That's a very common question. There is no pain associated with these procedures. Generally, there may be some minor soreness, which over-the-counter Tylenol or Advil can typically alleviate.

◇◇◇

QUESTION: Is there a simple, cost-effective solution to fix my discolored front teeth? How long would a procedure like this take?

ANSWER: We are happy to be able to offer an inexpensive and quick procedure to fix your tooth discoloration. Plus, we can do it in one visit. Some of our patients tell us that their smile makeover procedure has unexpectedly opened doors and opportunities. Whether you have a fast-approaching job interview or another event where you want to look your best, this procedure will give you the increased confidence that goes with a new smile.

QUESTION: Is there a fee to use your computer simulation technology?

ANSWER: As part of your initial consultation for your smile makeover, there is no fee for using our computer simulation software.

Free Offer

You deserve to find out more about your own smile makeover.

Imagine never having to worry about your teeth embarrassing you again. Picture not having to deal with painful teeth or pain in your mouth. Imagine no longer having to be self-conscious about your smile – never feeling a need to hide your smile.

Our entire team strives to make you feel as comfortable as possible in any treatment we provide here at *The Center for Dental Excellence.* Our high level of care and exceptional service starts the moment you walk in the door and never stops.

There is no obligation, so you really have nothing to lose. We invite you to schedule your appointment, come into our office, meet the team, and meet with one of our dentists. Schedule today while these consultations are 100% free by heading over to www.YourSmileMakeoverConsult.com or calling us at 708-866-0082.

Chapter 3

Dentures, Snap-In Dentures, Implants & All-On-4

Overview

If you're reading this chapter, chances are that your teeth are deteriorating, you're frustrated with your dentures, or you're simply living with pain in your mouth. Ultimately, we want to show that you don't have to suffer anymore. You can get back to living a normal life again.

Imagine what your life would be like if you never had to worry about your teeth falling out in public ever again. You'll never have to put your teeth in a glass or use paste or goo ever again. Take a moment and just visualize how it would feel if you had that smile you always wanted and could eat anything you wanted without trouble. Imagine how amazing that would feel.

In this chapter, we are going to show how you can easily have a complete new mouth. We will show how you can enjoy food again, improve your confidence, and even have an overall healthier life.

As we mentioned in the introduction, the timing is great right now for these procedures, because technology has evolved and improved significantly over the years. In addition, we have refined our skills and technique, because we've been performing the implant procedure at *The Center for Dental Excellence* since it was approved in the United States over 15 years ago.

We have been helping patients overcome struggles with dentures for over 25 years. In addition, we have developed our own unique system for the All-on-4 procedure with multiple doctors here at *The Center for Dental Excellence*. Finally, the materials available to you have improved greatly, making new teeth extremely durable today. Your implants are designed to be placed in your mouth once and last your lifetime.

We love helping our patients eliminate pain in their mouth and ill-fitting dentures. You can have a life without pain & ill-fitting dentures in as little as one day – guaranteed! We know you probably think that sounds too good to be true. This chapter is going to show exactly how we can make that happen.

In this chapter, you will learn:

- The myths and misconceptions about dentures, implants, and replacing both your upper and lower teeth in as little as a day;

- How new technology makes it likely that you can get dental implants now, even if you have been told in the past you weren't a candidate;

- How you'll gain confidence and a youthful smile – whether you're using dentures, getting dental implants, or replacing all of your teeth with the All-on-4 (a.k.a. "Teeth in a Day") procedure;

- How the process works for each of these procedures, as well as who can help you with these procedures.

By the end of this chapter, you will know exactly how to eliminate any painful dental conditions and – most importantly – be able to have teeth that will allow you to live better!

Why are we sharing this information with you? At *The Center for Dental Excellence,* we recognize that you have choices when it comes to your treatment. The goal of this chapter is to inform you about your options – from dentures to dental implants to the All-on-4 procedure. By explaining the variety of treatment options available today, we want to help you make the right decision for your unique needs.

12 Common Misconceptions about the All-on-4 Procedure and Dentures

---

Misconception #1: Age is a factor when getting dentures or having the All-on-4 procedure done.

Age is *definitely* not a factor. We have helped people of all ages with dentures and All-on-4, from young people to older people and everyone in between. Often, our patients express regret for waiting as long as they did to see us. The sooner you get your new custom- fitted dentures or All-on-4 procedure, the more years you can have to enjoy a better lifestyle.

Consider this: if you stop putting off your procedure, you will have many more years to enjoy your beautiful and healthy smile – *and* your procedure will cost less on a per-year basis. Options like bridges, crowns, and dentures typically only last 5 to 10 years. On the other hand, implants and the All-On-4 procedure are the most successful long-term solution for replacing missing teeth.

In short, age is not a factor, no matter what your age is.

◇◇◇

Misconception #2: The All-on-4 procedure must be painful.

Since we've been performing the All-on-4 procedure, most patients have not reported any serious pain. Some mention discomfort or minor swelling after the procedure, which is managed easily with over-the-counter medications like Advil or Tylenol.

The procedure itself is made very comfortable, thanks to

sedation. In addition, we ensure that you are in a comfortable environment while you are with us. From personal neck support pillows to warm blankets and more, our comfort menu will ensure your comfort throughout the entire procedure.

In fact, many people wake up from the procedure and ask, "When do we start?" That's when we get to tell them, "We are already finished. You have your new teeth!" We show them the mirror, and their excitement is palpable. Some of our patients report back to us that they are soon able to eat steak and anything else they want without issue!

◇◇◇

Misconception #3: Getting dentures will be painful if extractions are needed.

Each patient is given pain-relievers to minimize the pain or discomfort they may have. In one case, we had to remove all of a patient's teeth. He reported *no pain* during the procedure. All he needed was over-the-counter Tylenol, and he happily went to work the next day with his new smile.

◇◇◇

Misconception #4: You don't have enough bone for the All-on-4 procedure.

Have you already seen a dentist, an oral surgeon, or a periodontist who said you weren't a good candidate for implants because you didn't have enough bone? We're happy to tell you that times have changed! With this advanced technology, most people who come in to see us at *The Center for Dental Excellence* are in fact good candidates for the All-on-4 procedure without bone grafting.

◇◇◇

Misconception #5: You need one implant per tooth for the All-on-4.

This is not the case at all! The All-On-4 procedure is a state-of-the- art dental implant procedure that allows us to use only four implants for the entire upper or lower set of teeth, rather than having to use one implant per missing tooth. Just these four implants will allow you to chew like your natural teeth.

Misconception #6: You must go without teeth for a period of time if you want any of these procedures.

Some people think they'll have to go without teeth while their dentures are being made. While some dental offices will have you go a period of time without teeth, at *The Center for Dental Excellence* – regardless of your specific situation – you will *never* be without teeth.

If you opt for the All-On-4 procedure, you can also completely avoid temporary bridges, dentures, or going without teeth at all, which are common necessities during a standard dental implant procedure.

You will have a new set of fixed teeth the same day your implants are placed. The procedure usually takes only 3 to 4 hours. In addition to the short length of the procedure itself, many of our patients have also told us they needed almost no recovery time for their new teeth.

Imagine going home at the end of the day with a brand-new smile. Soon after your treatment, you will be free to eat your favorite foods again, laugh more, and smile more – just as you would with natural teeth.

Misconception #7: All-on-4 teeth require extra effort to care for them.

In fact, the All-on-4 dental implants are very easy to take care of. You simply treat them as you would natural teeth, with regular home care, dental check-ups, and professional cleanings.

Misconception #8: Implants can set off metal detectors at the airport.

Don't worry. They don't. You will be able to walk through metal detectors without needing any special accommodations.

◇◇◇

Misconception #9: These treatments are unaffordable.

This couldn't be further from the truth! First of all, many insurance plans cover the removal of teeth and even a portion of any subsequent procedure. At *The Center for Dental Excellence,* we will help make your treatment affordable by working with your insurance company to maximize your benefits.

In addition to using insurance, some of our patients have used their Health Savings or Flex Spending Accounts. We also have 0% financing plans available, and we accept all major credit cards to help make this procedure affordable for you. We have many affordability options that will fit your budget, and there may even be tax benefits for you.

It is also worth noting that the overall cost of the All-on-4 procedure is less when compared to single implants.

The fact is, everyone's circumstances are different, so the cost of dental implants will vary from case to case. The best way to get an accurate idea of what your dental implants will cost is to come in for your free consultation, which we'll discuss at the end of this chapter.

◇◇◇

Misconception #10: You must always use adhesive with dentures.

There are many denture options that do not require adhesives. Removable dentures, partial dentures, and snap-in-teeth (also known as denture stabilization) are all options where properly fitting dentures should not require adhesive to stay in place.

Also, with the customized, proper-fitting dentures that you get at *The Center for Dental Excellence,* those messy, gooey adhesives are rarely necessary for upper dentures. For people who are unable to wear their lower denture without adhesive, we offer many affordable solutions.

Misconception #11: If you have dentures, everyone will know it.

To demystify this misconception, we're going to share what one of our patients said: "People cannot believe these are false teeth! That shows you what a good job he did."

Indeed, denture materials have evolved exponentially over the years. When they are fitted properly, you simply cannot tell that dentures are false teeth anymore.

Misconception #12: All dentures are the same.

You might as well say apples and oranges are the same! When you compare plain, regular dentures to the custom dentures we make at *The Center for Dental Excellence,* you'll discover many differences. For example:

- **You'll enjoy the highest quality materials *and* teeth.**

- **Your dentures will have a proper fit.**

- **Our unique customization process will include your own prototype,** which allows you to preview what your new teeth will feel like.

- **You'll enjoy our high-level service** – our beautiful office, your welcome gift, our knowledgeable and friendly staff, the easy parking, the warm towels when you're done with your appointment, the convenient location, your comfort menu, and the available refreshments. In the same way that we pay attention to every detail when it comes to your dentures, we also care about your comfort, which can make a huge difference in your overall dental experience.

- At *The Center for Dental Excellence,* we provide a

100% satisfaction guarantee.

- With our conventional dentures, we include **lifetime check-ups and adjustments.**

- **We make your custom dentures affordable.** Many dental insurances cover the cost of any teeth removal, as well as the cost of the dentures themselves, and we will work to ensure you get the best coverage possible. We also have some patients who have used their Health Savings or Flex Spending Accounts.

We have 0% financing plans available, and we accept all major credit cards. We recognize that everyone's budget is different. We will work with you, so you can get the smile you desire and deserve. The best way to get an accurate idea of what your dentures will cost is to come in for your free consultation.

Your Options

For those of you who are missing or will be missing all of your teeth, you have four main options. The first option is the All-on-4 procedure, where new teeth are fixed in your mouth to function like your own natural teeth. The second option is to get dentures that snap into places using implants. Your third option is to get removable, custom, cosmetic dentures. Finally, your last option is to do nothing at all.

◇◇◇

All-on-4

The All-on-4 procedure places four titanium implants in such a way that the bone will envelop and secure them into place. The implants placed in the back part of the jaw are angulated to achieve maximum advantage with the existing bone.

There are very few health issues that would keep a patient from having this procedure done, and virtually all people we see for this procedure are candidates. In order for us to properly evaluate and plan your case, you will initially require a consultation and diagnostic appointment. These initial steps allow us to present you with all the alternatives, so that we can decide together the best treatment based on your individual needs and wants.

Like in everything, technology has changed in our lives, and it has improved the way that we can transform your smile. We now use modern technology to obtain essential information about your mouth and jaw, such as a diagnosis of the amount of bone you have. Then we can customize your treatment accordingly. We use a CT scan, which gives us a 360-degree and 3-dimensional view of your bone, allowing us to perform a guided, minimally invasive procedure. Even if you have previously been told that you can't have dental implants, chances are that you really can.

When you decide to move forward with the treatment, the implants will be placed and the new replacement teeth fitted all in one day. Because only four implants are used in the procedure, the entire process takes much less of your time and is more affordable than previous treatments.

Remember, your teeth are permanent and fixed, so there is no need for you to be without teeth or to endure temporary removable dentures for an extended time period. You can come in for a morning appointment and leave that same afternoon with a brand new, radiant smile!

◇◇◇

Snap-in Dentures and Custom-fit Dentures

If you presently have a denture that was made years ago, we can now not only improve the look of your teeth, but also give you a facelift-like result as well. We can reduce wrinkles, improve your profile, and give you a more natural, youthful appearance.

Our dentures are natural-looking, removable replacement teeth. At *The Center for Dental Excellence,* we fabricate the dentures to custom-fit your unique mouth, helping you to avoid adhesives or messy pastes. If you have some healthy teeth remaining, you may be a candidate for a partial denture. Those are customized in the same way as full dentures.

When it comes to the process of dentures, there are a few simple steps. We start by taking an impression of your mouth. On subsequent visits, we'll make more impressions with finer details. From those, we then fashion a customized prototype of the denture for your unique mouth. This allows you to have a preview of your new and improved smile.

After your prototype is approved, we have the dentures custom-made. During the initial fitting, your new dentures will first be tried in your mouth, and you'll then wear them until your next visit. We will make any necessary adjustments to ensure they fit as well and as comfortably as possible.

For Snap-In Dentures, we place two to four titanium implants in the upper or lower jaw. A customized, cosmetic denture is fabricated with snaps inside. This allows the denture to snap securely onto the implants, providing more stability and bringing you more comfort and better chewing abilities. Your dentures literally snap into place with this method. Believe it or not, this can be done in one day!

Once you have your dentures and they start to become part of your everyday life, you should still visit us once a year for a checkup. This way, we can make sure your oral health is in the best possible shape. We can also make sure you're getting the very best out of your dentures and that they continue to fit properly.

Doing Nothing

This is your fourth available option if you are missing some or all of your teeth. Look at what happens if you don't replace them. As in the picture on the left with no teeth, your face collapses in. If left untreated longer, the face collapses even more, like in the second picture. Finally, in the picture on the right, you can see how all of our treatment options give support to your face, providing a much more youthful appearance.

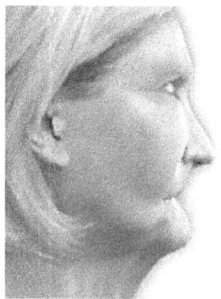 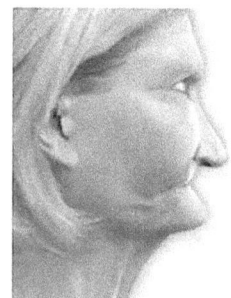 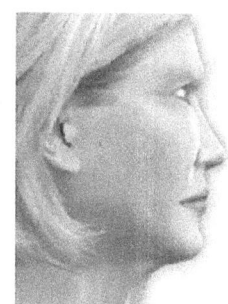

Choosing the Best Option for You

We invite you to talk with us at *The Center for Dental Excellence*. We have extensive training and experience with the All-on-4 procedure, implants, and dentures. We would love the chance to talk more about your specific mouth and treatment options, so together we can customize a plan for your unique needs and desires.

Life-Changing Stories

The Mayo Clinic performed a study that showed people who have their teeth live longer, healthier lives compared to those who struggle with dentures. Therefore, there is truth to the notion that healthier teeth can lead to an overall healthier life.

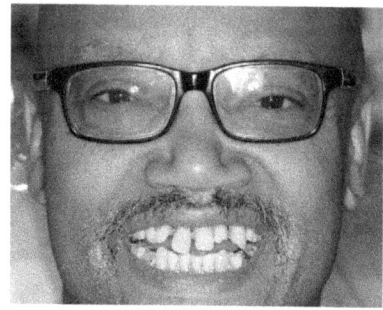

Take, for example, a patient of ours who was doing a lot of talking during his workday. His teeth would start to slip because he was using adhesive with his partial. After having us perform the All-on-4 procedure, he told us, "Now I have no problems! I actually smile when I take pictures." He doesn't need to make adjustments when he eats anymore, either. "I never could eat an apple before without cutting it up," he said. "Now I take the apple and bite right into it."

Up on the right, you can see the "before" picture of another patient. After learning about the All-on-4 procedure, he knew he wanted to proceed with it.

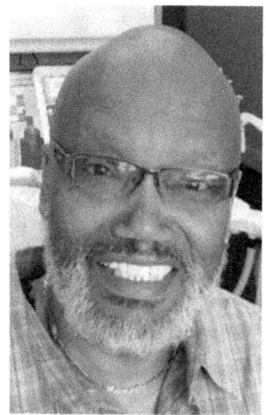

Now look at this "after" photograph. Our patient reported no difficulties with any part of the treatment, and he is very satisfied with the results.

As you can imagine when you compare these two photos, the All-on-4 procedure improved our patient's life dramatically. He's received compliments on his smile from family and friends. He's thrilled to have control over his diet – to have a choice in what he eats and how he gets to eat it. Now, he says, he would recommend the procedure to anyone and everyone, declaring that "this has changed my life very much for the better."

This next patient's biggest fear was that the treatment would be painful. When she was finished, she expressed how happy she was with the experience: "I am glad to say there wasn't any pain at all. From the time I entered *The Center for Dental Excellence* office, everyone has been so friendly, knowledgeable, and 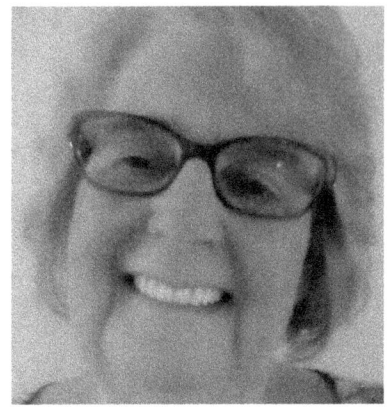 concerned for my comfort and well-being. I have been so pleased and satisfied with the outcome. It has given me the confidence to smile again. I have a better overall feeling about myself. The treatment has been the best I've ever had, from the standpoint of how everything falls into place as far as fitting and convenience, looking and feeling better than my natural teeth, which I never thought I would have again. I can honestly say I am so glad I chose to have this done."

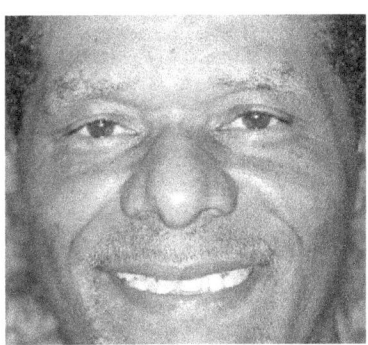 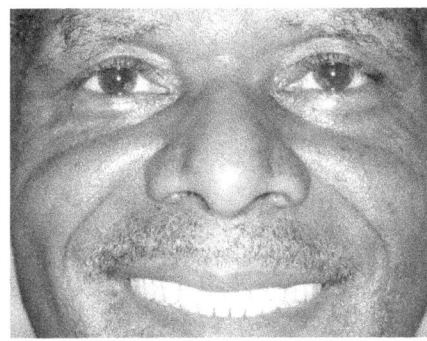

Another patient of ours had horrible infections in his mouth that were causing his overall health to deteriorate. Sometimes he had trouble even getting out of bed and going to work. His condition was getting worse, and he couldn't afford treatment.

Thankfully, his sister decided to cover the investment of the All-on-4 procedure. When you compare his "before" and "after" pictures on the previous page, you can see not only a healthier smile, but also a healthier, happier patient.

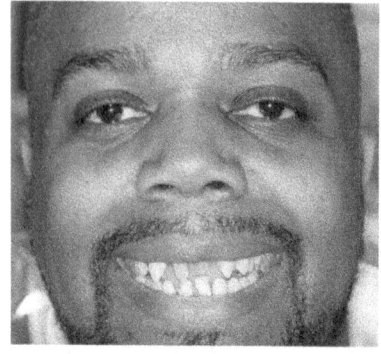

Here is a patient who on one hand thought, "I'm too young to lose all my teeth and be like my grandma!" On the other hand, he realized he was also too young to be suffering with such unhealthy teeth and gums. He had a disease that needed to be treated.

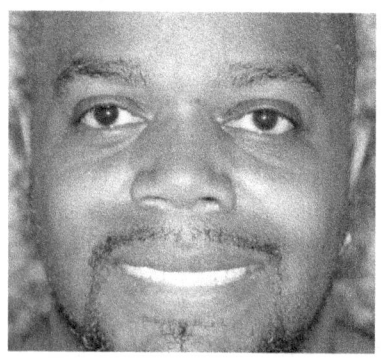

Before the procedure, he had multiple health issues. He wasn't sleeping well, didn't smile much, and experienced significant pain, especially in the winter when cold air would hit his teeth. In fact, it was a struggle even to get him to smile for this "before" picture. He was embarrassed of his missing teeth and how his smile looked.

We fitted him for upper and lower dentures. Afterward, he reported that he had *no pain*. He felt younger and more confident. He was smiling much more readily. Equally important, his energy was back, and he was able to complete projects. His social life even improved!

"Not only would I recommend the procedure to other people," he said, "I would have done it much sooner. Natural teeth are overrated. These feel like second nature to me. The people at *The Center for Dental Excellence* didn't just take good care of me, they took GREAT care of me. I loved every single minute of my time there and am very thankful I found them."

The feeling is definitely mutual. We're very grateful that he found us, so we could help him with this life-changing transformation. When, you look at his "before" and "after" pictures side by side, you see a completely different person in the "after" photograph. His whole face and demeanor has changed.

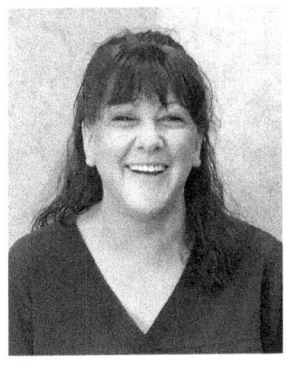

This next patient is a nurse who came to us for an upper denture and lower overdenture (also known as the snap-in denture). We used two implants to secure her lower denture.

When she first came to our office, she told us she was absolutely "petrified" because of unpleasant experiences with prior dentists. We spoke with her at length about the procedure and helped put her mind at ease.

After the procedure, she was utterly thrilled with her new smile. It was life changing for her to even be able to smile. She could eat anything she wanted, and she could even chew gum! She says her life has improved simply from knowing she can smile and laugh without covering her mouth in embarrassment. She enjoys her newfound outgoing nature, too, now that she doesn't feel ashamed of her smile. She happily tells friends and family that *The Center for Dental Excellence* is the place that can help them with their smiles, too.

At this point, we want to share some more stories from patients who have improved their smiles and lifestyles with our custom dentures.

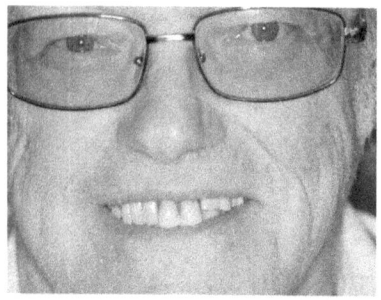

This patient was initially worried about the amount of time involved with his procedure and how his body would heal. Overall, he was nervous about the unknown – a completely understandable feeling for anyone about to undergo a life-changing procedure. He said that speaking with the doctor and our entire team really put him at ease.

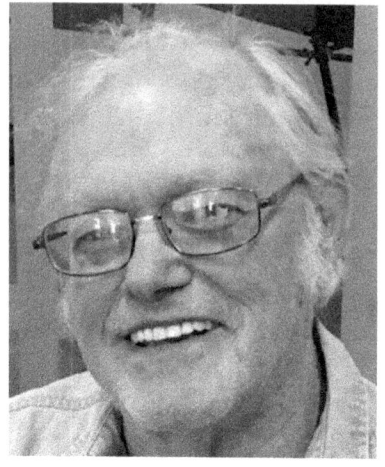

Just look at his "after" picture (on the next page) compared to his "before." He told us that he is beyond happy that he did this for himself. He's thrilled with the way his teeth look, and now he can even eat corn on the cob with his new dentures! He loves getting compliments on his smile from people, and he is constantly referring people to our office. When you examine his before and after pictures side-by-side, you can see how natural his new teeth look.

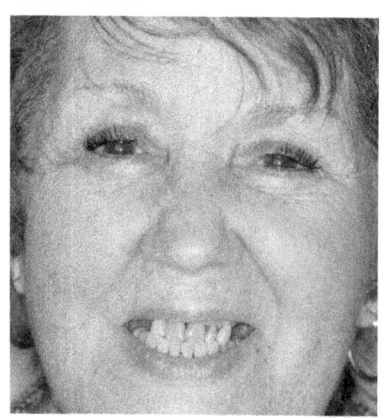

This final patient we'd like to discuss was searching for a new dentist for quite a long time. She took the advice and recommendations of others, but she never found one that she felt was the right fit until the day she met Dr. Goldberg and our staff at *The Center for Dental Excellence.* She immediately felt at ease with everyone. She felt welcome, as though she was part of a family.

Here you see her "before" picture, and her "after" picture with her new upper denture is on the next page.

She is happier with the results than she ever imagined she could be. She receives compliments all the time on how natural her teeth look. In addition, like the previous patient we described, she gets to eat whatever she wants – even corn on the cob!

Once again, look at her new teeth in her "after" photo. They look like her own, *natural* teeth!

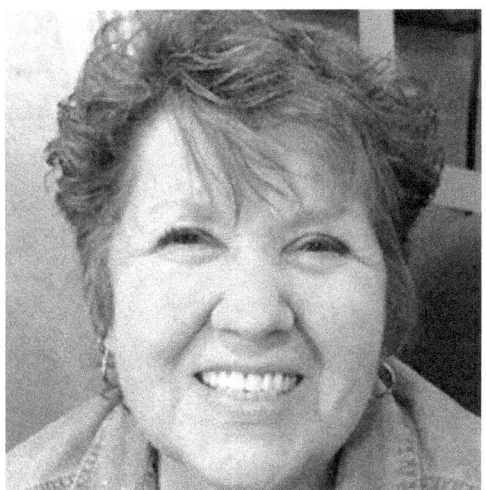

This patient and the rest of her family all come to *The Center for Dental Excellence* now for all their dental care, and they continue to spread the word about the great works and caring professionals at our office.

We could share countless stories about people whose lives have been changed for the better by the All-on-4 procedure and by dentures, but here's an even better idea: why don't you become our next success story?

Your Most Common Questions Answered

QUESTION: Compared to dentures, what is the roof of the mouth like after the All-on-4 procedure?

ANSWER: It may amaze you to learn that the roof of your mouth is not covered at all when you opt for the All-on-4 procedure! There is no acrylic or plastic top like with your dentures. You will regain the taste and sensation of food.

◇◇◇

QUESTION: Because of my dentures, I make embarrassing clicking sounds while speaking and eating. The dentures have clearly affected my speech. Will the All-on-4 procedure help improve my speech and stop these clicking sounds?

ANSWER: Absolutely! The All-on-4 procedure allows for a more permanent and stronger hold than dentures. This typically causes those clicking sounds to go away. Many patients have reported back to us that a previous speech problem no longer exists. However, before we recommend the All-on-4 procedure or any other alternatives, we invite you to come in for an evaluation of your current dentures. We may be able to make some adjustments to improve their overall fit, and sometimes that will help the clicking sound to go away.

◇◇◇

QUESTION: Another dentist told me I don't have enough bone for implants. Should I still come and see you?

ANSWER: You should definitely come to our office. You probably *do* have enough bone, and we can use a state-of-the art CT scan to confirm whether that is indeed true.

QUESTION: How long will these implants last?

ANSWER: With proper care, your implants can last a lifetime.

◇◇◇

QUESTION: How long do dentures typically last? Do I still need to see a dentist after I get my dentures?

ANSWER: With proper care, dentures can typically last ten years or even longer. That said, you should still come see your dentist at least once a year for regular checkups. We want to make sure your dentures are still fitting properly, and we'll check your overall gum and mouth health. We also check for oral cancer. For our denture patients, these annual checks are free for a lifetime.

◇◇◇

QUESTION: Will insurance cover my treatment plan?

ANSWER: Many dental insurance companies and some medical insurances help to defray the cost of implant treatment. We also have interest- free financing and flexible payment plan options, and we accept all major credit cards. As with any treatment here at *The Center for Dental Excellence,* we have many affordable options to fit every budget.

◇◇◇

QUESTION: What does an implant look like?

ANSWER: An implant looks like the root of a tooth. When you come in for your consultation, we'll show you exactly what an implant looks like.

◇◇◇

QUESTION: Are there any health issues that would prevent me from having the All-on-4 procedure?

ANSWER: We have helped many people with the All-on-4 procedure, including patients with diabetes, high blood pressure, osteoporosis, and other health complications. As long as your diabetes is controlled, you can still be a candidate. There are extremely limited conditions that would prevent you from having this procedure. We always work closely with your medical provider to ensure your safety and health.

QUESTION: The All-on-4 procedure and the dentures process both seem so simple. Are they really that straightforward?

ANSWER: With the advanced technology we have in our office, these procedures *are* relatively simple. Since each patient is unique to us, we find it best to go over the technical aspects and details of your specific procedure when you come to see us for your consultation.

QUESTION: Do I need a referral from a specialist to come and see you?

ANSWER: No referral is required, although many of our patients are referred to us from a friend, a family member, or another doctor. We are always happy to give second opinions as well.

QUESTION: Is there an age where you won't perform either of these procedures?

ANSWER: Age is not an important factor in determining whether you are a candidate. We have patients in their late 80s and even 90s who have received implants.

QUESTION: What is the success rate of the All-on-4 procedure?

ANSWER: We have an overall 95% success rate with the procedure.

QUESTION: My denture cracked. Can you repair my dentures, or do I need new ones?

ANSWER: Because we have a laboratory on the premises, we are able to repair most dentures with great accuracy and speed while you wait. We should be able to repair your dentures very easily.

QUESTION: I need the rest of my teeth taken out, and I need dentures. I'm worried about having to take time off from work. After I get my teeth taken out, how long does it take to get my new dentures?

ANSWER: Great news! You will get your dentures the same day you have your teeth removed. You'll be able to go to work the next day.

Free Offer

Imagine never having to worry about your teeth falling out again. Picture not having to deal with tooth pain or pain in your mouth. Imagine never having to worry about paste or goo ever again. And best of all, imagine never feeling self-conscious about your smile.

We invite you to take the next step toward making all that a reality. Schedule a thorough consultation and examination at *The Center for Dental Excellence*, during which we can assess your unique mouth and confirm that you're a good candidate for dentures, implants, or the All-on-4.

During this initial consultation, we'll also talk about the custom cosmetic enhancements that we can perform for you with these procedures. For example, you may want whiter teeth. You may want to eliminate some wrinkles. Maybe you want to look younger. Maybe you want to look more masculine or more feminine, or maybe you want to eat better. Maybe it's all about a better self-image or simply about being healthier by being able to eat healthier foods. When you come to *The Center for Dental Excellence,* we aren't just replacing your teeth. We're helping you improve your lifestyle.

Keep in mind: our free consultation is *not* for you if you're not open-minded to new technologies. This also isn't for you if you are not willing to invest in improving your health, your confidence, or your new smile.

On the other hand, our free consultation *is* for you if you want to discover your best treatment option. This is also for you if you want a healthier smile. Ultimately, our complimentary evaluation is for you if you want to live a confident, more fulfilled life.

There's no obligation. You really have nothing to lose! We invite you to schedule your appointment, come into our office, meet our team, and consult with one of our dentists. We urge you to schedule today while these consultations are 100% free, too! To do this, go to www.YourFreeAllOn4Consult.com or call us at (708) 866-0063.

Ultimately, our entire team strives to make you feel as comfortable as possible during any treatment we provide here at *The Center for Dental Excellence.* Our high level of care and exceptional service starts the moment you walk in the door and never stops.

Chapter 4

Sleep Apnea Solved Without a CPAP Machine

Overview

Do you have a CPAP machine or been told that you need one? If you do, you've most likely been diagnosed with sleep apnea. Sleep apnea is a very serious condition with numerous negative side effects and impacts on your medical health, including high blood pressure and an increased risk for heart attacks.

Are you snoring or waking up gasping and choking at night? Maybe you're experiencing heartburn or acid reflux (also known as GERD). Most likely, you don't feel refreshed in the morning; instead, you wake up still tired. Many people have reported having car accidents or near misses because of how tired they feel even after a full night's sleep.

If this is you, you are not alone. Many people continue to suffer even after being diagnosed with sleep apnea, because they don't or can't use their CPAP machine. Plus, most alternatives to a CPAP machine are more aggressive and irreversible – if they even work for you at all.

Now imagine what your life would be like if you never had to use your CPAP machine again – and could still feel more energetic and well-rested. Picture waking up refreshed and having more energy. How amazing would that be?

In this chapter, we'll discuss a new sleep appliance that can positively change your life. It's called *oral appliance therapy.* People are more compliant with oral appliance therapy because the device is far more comfortable and easy to use than a CPAP machine. Many of our patients say their spouses are even sleeping better, because their sleep is no longer being disturbed by snoring or the loud CPAP machine.

Here is what we'll review as we discuss oral appliance therapy in this chapter:

- Some of the myths and misconceptions about sleep appliances;
- How you can sleep better again by using oral appliance therapy;
- How the process works for getting your own sleep appliance, so you won't need your CPAP machine any longer;
- What you need to do so that oral appliance therapy can be covered by your insurance plan.

By the end of this chapter, you will be educated about this new alternative to your CPAP machine, and you will know exactly how to get a good night's rest again.

3 Misconceptions about Sleep Apnea

Misconception #1: Oral appliance therapy is difficult to get used to when you're trying to sleep.

To address this misconception, let us share a story about one of our patients.

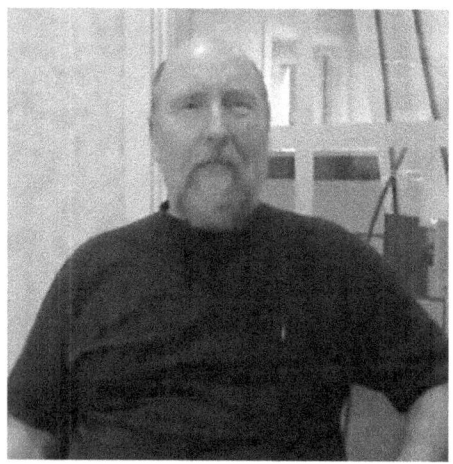

This patient of Dr. Greenebaum's tried pillows, but they didn't work. He tried the CPAP machine with a nasal attachment, but it caused his mouth to open and woke him up. He tried the full-mask CPAP machine, but he couldn't take all the pressure. In addition, the machine's noise kept him awake. He just couldn't fall asleep using a CPAP machine.

Eventually, he came to our office for oral appliance therapy. It worked instantly. He stopped snoring. Nothing caused him to wake up. Instead, he enjoyed a restful sleep that lasted the entire night. In his own words:

"After a month of using the appliance, I had another sleep study, and I passed the sleep study with no apneas. It was awesome! For me, I am a commercial truck driver, I needed that to be able to continue to be doing my job. This was extremely critical for me. And I can take this appliance anywhere I want to go. I put it in my briefcase and I go all across the country. Not a problem.

I no longer have to take a big machine. It works awesome, I love it, and my wife loves it."

Think about what he said – the sleep appliance worked *instantly*. Oral appliance therapy is like wearing a simple mouth guard, and it is incredibly easy to get used to.

Misconception #2: Oral appliance therapy is expensive.

If you have a copy of your sleep study and a referral from a physician, then we can get this new appliance covered by your medical insurance in almost all cases. Additionally, we offer flexible payment plans and 0% financing if you don't have any insurance.

Misconception #3: Sleep apnea only affects older people.

While sleep apnea is more common for people over the age of 40, it can strike anyone at any age, even children. If you think you or a loved one has sleep apnea, you should see a physician and request a diagnosis. A sleep study can rule out this potentially fatal condition. If the study shows that you do suffer from sleep apnea, however, we can use the sleep study and physician referral to help you get the oral appliance therapy you need.

Oral Appliance Therapy: Your Alternative to CPAP

By now you're likely wondering: what exactly *is* oral appliance therapy? Oral appliance therapy is a mouthpiece for patients with primary snoring or mild to moderate sleep apnea. It is completely non-invasive. The small device, which you wear while you sleep, is similar in size to an orthodontic retainer or a sports mouthguard. It is very comfortable, simple to wear, and easy to bring with you when you travel.

Oral appliances work by moving the jaw forward. This prevents the collapse of the tongue and soft tissues in the back of your throat, thereby keeping your airway open to allow adequate air intake. Oral appliance therapy involves selecting an appropriate design and then custom fitting it to your teeth. It can be used alone or in conjunction with other treatments.

Life-Changing Stories

Oral appliance therapy has changed the lives of so many of our patients, and it can change yours, too. Just consider what one of our patients said about his experience:

"It really works! I have been able to sleep comfortably. I sleep the whole time. My wife is happy. She no longer has to sleep in another room because I am no longer snoring too loud. It's a real tranquil sleep."

At this point, we want to share more testimonials from patients who have used this appliance.

"I was referred by a sleep doctor to *The Center for Dental Excellence* for a dental appliance to treat my sleep apnea. I could not have been sent to a better place. They patiently explained my treatment and monitored my progress while slowly advancing the oral appliance to gently open my airway at night and not compromise or change my bite. I consider myself very fortunate to be in the care of *The Center for Dental Excellence.* There are very few providers for this appliance in our area, and their service is excellent."

"I was diagnosed with sleep apnea. I have been using my sleep appliance for about a week. I no longer have to use caffeine during the day, whereas I had to before. Now, I don't get that exhausted feeling. It really has made a difference in my alertness level and my quality of life."

"For many years, I have woken up not feeling refreshed. Originally, I had attributed this to allergies. Some friends referred me to *The Center for Dental Excellence* to help understand my options regarding sleep appliances. After getting my dental appliance, I felt significantly better the first morning I woke up. I'm not having any discomfort, and I'm sleeping much better and waking up more refreshed. I would definitely recommend *The Center for Dental Excellence* if you are having snoring problems and to see if you might be a candidate for a sleep appliance."

You owe it to yourself and deserve to find out if you would be a good candidate for this life-changing sleep appliance. Imagine no longer having to worry about getting a good night's rest. Imagine no longer worrying about keeping your spouse awake or having to use your CPAP machine. With oral appliance therapy, this can all become a reality.

Your Most Common Questions Answered

QUESTION: I currently don't have dental insurance. Will my medical insurance cover oral appliance therapy?

ANSWER: Yes, your medical insurance will typically cover this appliance if you have a sleep study and a referral from your physician. Our team here at *The Center for Dental Excellence* can help you with the insurance paperwork to ensure you get the maximum benefit.

◇◇◇

QUESTION: Why is it so important to get my sleep apnea treated?

ANSWER: There are two main reasons to treat snoring and apnea.

The first reason is to improve your quality of life. Sleep is critical for your body's healing process and your ability to perform normally throughout the day. Apnea and snoring, on the other hand, can result in altered sleep patterns that undermine your body's healing functions. Snoring, of course, can also be a nuisance to a bed partner.

The second reason involves the relationship between apnea and numerous serious medical consequences. Untreated sleep apnea can cause or worsen many conditions, such as high blood pressure, heart attack, stroke, impotency, depression, and diabetes, to name just a few.

◇◇◇

QUESTION: What exactly IS oral appliance therapy?

ANSWER: An oral appliance is a small device, similar to an orthodontic retainer or an athletic mouthguard, which you wear in your mouth during sleep. Some oral appliances hold the lower jaw forward during sleep, preventing your throat tissues and tongue from collapsing, while others have a direct effect on tongue position. Fabricating an oral appliance is comfortable and non-invasive.

QUESTION: How do I know if an oral sleep appliance can help me?

ANSWER: After a comprehensive examination and review of your sleep study, we'll determine if you are a candidate for an oral appliance. Once the appliance is custom-made for your mouth, it will be slowly adjusted to maximize its capabilities.

Success may come instantly, with results obvious in as little as one night. In some cases, it may take several adjustments to reach a healthy outcome. No medical treatment, including CPAP, surgery, or oral appliance therapy, can guarantee that your apnea will be eliminated, but the only way to treat apnea is to try one of these treatments.

◊◊◊

QUESTION: How effective is oral appliance therapy?

ANSWER: Although oral appliances do not work on everybody, a well-made, well-fitted appliance will reduce or eliminate snoring. In most cases, the appliance will also significantly relieve or even eliminate the symptoms of sleep apnea. According to literature and clinical trials, oral appliance therapy is 84.0% effective in treatment of non-severe Obstructive Sleep Apnea cases and 69.2% effective for severe cases.

◊◊◊

QUESTION: How long will the sleep appliance last?

ANSWER: This is a new treatment option, so long-term data has not been confirmed yet. We tell our patients to estimate that their appliance will last 3-5 years, although we expect many will last much longer, possibly even up to 10 years. Patients with heavy bruxing (tooth-grinding) activity may wear out their appliances faster.

QUESTION: How long does it take to get the appliance?

ANSWER: If you decide to proceed with oral appliance therapy at your first office visit, we can take impressions immediately and then schedule your appliance insertion visit. Usually that appointment can be scheduled within a few weeks of your initial visit.

QUESTION: How can I be sure the appliance is effective once I've been fitted?

ANSWER: Once you have had two weeks of better sleep while wearing the device, we will refer you back to your physician. He or she can then confirm the effectiveness of the appliance.

QUESTION: Can this sleep appliance work for people without teeth?

ANSWER: Yes! Depending on the type of appliance and the condition of your mouth, an oral appliance can be made for people without teeth.

Free Offer

How will your life be if you don't learn more about this new sleep appliance? What will life be like if you don't use your CPAP machine or do nothing about your sleep apnea? How will you feel in the morning? Will the snoring affect other people? Will it jeopardize your job? How will this affect you mentally, physically, and, of course, emotionally?

This is where we here at *The Center for Dental Excellence* can help you. Simply head over to www.YourBetterSleepConsult.com or call us at (708) 866-0126 to schedule your no-obligation, free consultation with one of our highly trained and trusted doctors. During your appointment, we will answer all your questions, educate you further about the sleep appliance, and see if you would be a good candidate.

Now this free consultation may *not* be for you if you're satisfied with your CPAP or if you're not interested in improving your health. On the other hand, this free consultation is definitely for you if you're open-minded to a new type of appliance that you can easily wear while you sleep. This *is* for you if you want a better night's sleep and improved health without using an uncomfortable CPAP machine.

Ultimately, our team strives to make you feel as comfortable as possible with every treatment we provide at *The Center for Dental Excellence.* Our high level of care and exceptional service starts the moment you walk in the door and never ends. We want you to feel better, get better sleep, and ultimately live better. Patients tell us all the time that this sleep appliance is a life-changing device for them. They tell us they can once again sleep peacefully and wake well-rested. We want you to have that same transformation, so contact us today to schedule your free consultation.

Chapter 5

Your Next Step

What Is the Next Step?

We have done our best to fill this book with as much valuable information as possible. Now that you have been educated on the wide variety of treatment options available to you, you may find yourself asking two logical questions: Of all these treatments, which is best for you? And what should you do next? We'll address the second question first: *What should you do next?*

At this point, you really have two options:

Option #1:

You could do nothing and probably continue to hide your smile – or maybe smile without showing your teeth. If you are currently in pain, then doing nothing will mostly likely cause your pain to get worse.

Let's face it. The option of doing nothing doesn't make much sense. You do not have to live with pain or hide your smile any longer.

Option #2:

For your second option, we invite you to speak with us or another one of the dentists at *The Center for Dental Excellence*. We are all highly trained and experienced with every procedure discussed throughout this book, and we can determine which treatment plans or procedures make the most sense for you. We'd love the chance to talk more about your specific mouth and options. Together, we can customize a plan for your unique needs and desires.

How to Schedule an Appointment

To schedule an appointment with us, simply head over to www.YourFreeDentalConsult.com or call us at (708) 866-0063 to schedule your initial visit.

Your initial visit is normally $249. However, if you mention this book when you call or fill out the form at www.YourFreeDentalConsult.com, you will get a comprehensive examination with x-rays and a complete treatment consultation completely free. This is a $249 value with no obligation.

We're making this offer because we want to make it easy for you to see us. We want you to have a risk-free opportunity to find out if we are the right dental office for you.

During your initial visit, we will listen to your questions and concerns, perform an examination with x-rays, and generate any necessary computer models. If helpful, we will also use our computer-generated imaging technology to show you what is possible for your smile. Remember, we offer same-day resolution on many procedures as well. In other words, if we mutually determine that a procedure or treatment is right for you, we can most likely begin your treatment on the same day as your initial visit.

Patient Reviews

Let us leave you with a few final examples of patients whose lives were changed by visiting *The Center for Dental Excellence.*

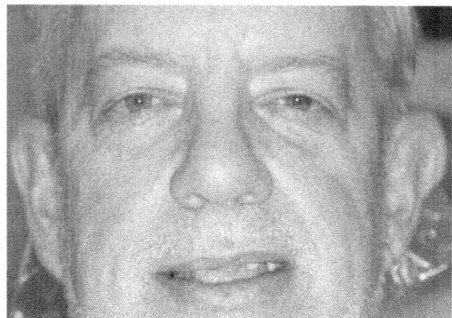

This is a "before" of one of our patients. He did a complete smile makeover using a combination of the treatments discussed in this book.

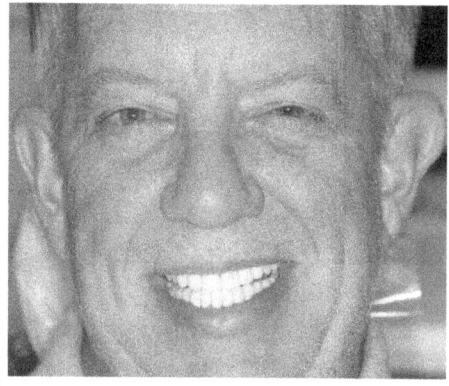

Now look at his amazing "after" photo. Not only does he have renewed confidence and self-esteem, but now he can also eat the foods he wants with ease. This is something he hasn't been able to do in years. When you compare his two photos, you can easily see his improved demeanor and new youthful smile.

This next patient had orthodontic treatment through a specialist, but she still had not achieved her ideal smile. This was easily corrected the same day with a minor bonding procedure. When you look at the "before" and "after" photos side-by-side here, you can clearly see a more beautiful, finished look to her teeth.

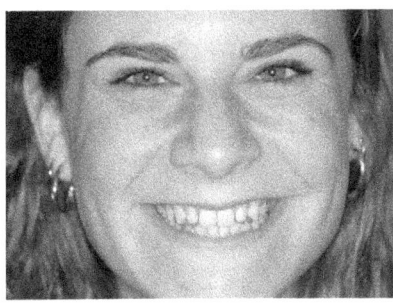 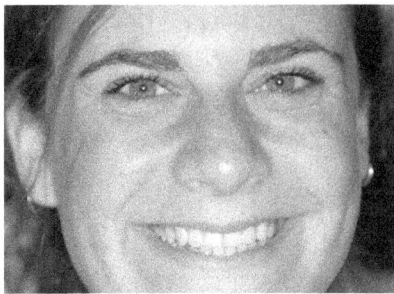

The husband of this next patient had his smile makeover first. It resulted in his smiling more and looking more handsome – but now he looked about 15 years younger than she did! She came in to see us and said, "I don't want to look like my husband's mother any more. What can we do?" We showed her the Smile Vision workup of her smile, and she was amazed.

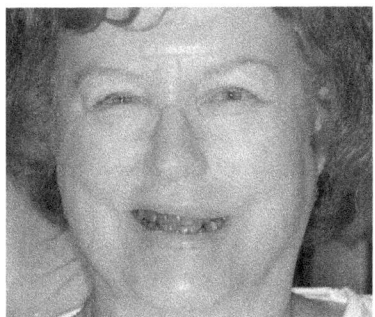 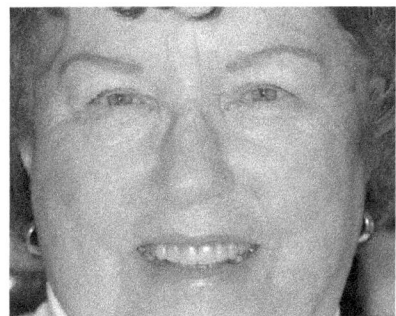

Compare her "before" and "after" pictures. She reports that not a single person has asked if she had her teeth redone. Instead, everyone *does* approach her to comment on her attractive, youthful appearance.

Here is her experience in her own words: "Before you say 'no way' to your mouth looking sensational, I will say that I will never have to see dental specialists or have teeth pulled. None of mine were ever pulled, and I had not one bit of pain. I am transformed for LIFE. I always have smiled, as I am a happy person – but, though I was a skeptic, magical things have happened to my work life, my home life, and it is a lot more fun to look in the mirror. I am dazzling! The price of the million-dollar smile has been priceless to my life and my world...and two years ago, I would not have believed I would be saying that – EVER! So, with that, I recommend you not just strongly consider a smile makeover for yourself, but you simply come in and talk with a dentist at *The Center for Dental Excellence* and they will make it happen."

Now this next patient also had a smile makeover. She has gone to a hygienist at a periodontist's office for many years. After our patient's makeover, her hygienist (who looks at people's teeth every day) said she has never seen such high-quality work. She told the patient she can always tell who has seen one of our dentists at *The Center for Dental Excellence.* Here are the "before" and computer-generated pictures for that patient:

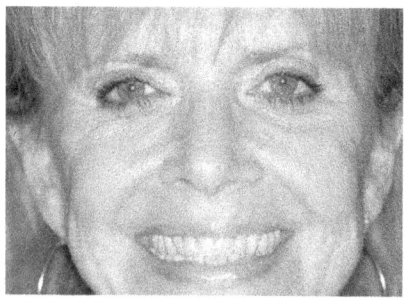 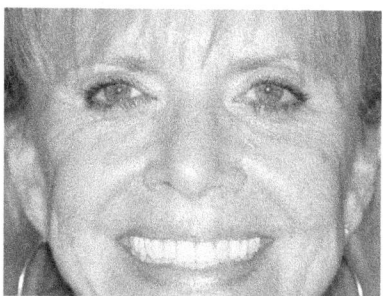

And here is her "after" picture:

She reported back that the treatment was never uncomfortable – not once. She had no tooth aches, not even after gum surgery. It was all *so* worth it. She feels younger. She has a big smile, so her teeth really show. People still compliment her and notice her beautiful teeth – even strangers!

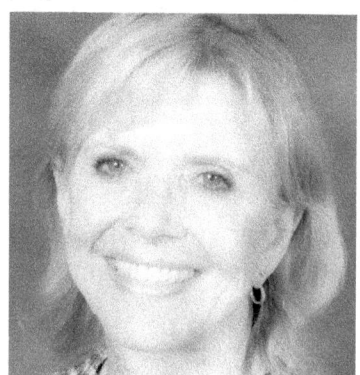

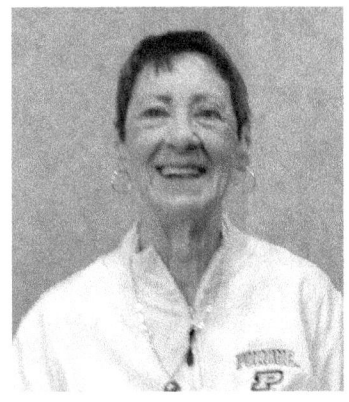

This next patient had an upper denture and lower overdenture, which is also known as the snap-in denture. We used two implants to secure the lower denture.

She has worn a complete upper denture since she was 18 years old. At one time, she had most of her lower teeth and a fixed bridge. Some years back, she had problems with a rear tooth that another dentist had "screwed up," and everything went "downhill from there."

She left that dentist and came to *The Center for Dental Excellence*. We recommended new upper and lower dentures. She followed our advice and was very pleased with the results.

We recreated her smile for her, and she began to feel much better, both physically and emotionally. She then decided to move forward with two lower implants to help support and retain her lower denture. She is thrilled with those results, too. She feels like her teeth are a natural part of her body again, and she knows that she made the right decision. When friends and family are considering a dentist to treat them, she recommends them to us wholeheartedly.

Your Free Offer

To schedule your consultation, visit our website at www.YourFreeDentalConsult.com or simply call us at (708) 866-0063.

There is no obligation and this consultation is 100% free.

We want you to feel better, look better and ultimately live better. Patients tell us all the time that coming to see us is a life-changing experience for them. They tell us they can once again talk, laugh, and eat comfortably with family, friends, and co-workers. They no longer feel held hostage by their teeth.

We want you to have that same transformation, so contact us today to schedule your free consultation. We look forward to seeing you very soon!

Endorsements

Here's What Professionals Have to Say About The Center for Dental Excellence!

As the founder of one the premier dental laboratories in America, I consider myself fortunate to work with Drs. Cary N. Goldberg and Charles J. Greenebaum. We work with the best of the best across the nation and these doctors have earned a position on that list with every case they send us. Not only are they among the top cosmetic dentists in the south suburbs, but their expertise runs far deeper than just a beautiful smile. Dr. Goldberg's and Dr. Greenebaum's knowledge of implants, full-mouth reconstruction, and sleep medicine show a focus on total oral health and overall wellbeing far beyond that of the average dentist. As an added bonus, they work with one of the most talented teams in group practice at The Center for Dental Excellence.

Luke Kahng, President
LSK 121 Oral Prosthetics
Naperville, IL

The South Suburban area is fortunate to have a highly knowledgeable, skilled, compassionate group of dentists, headed by Dr. Charles Greenebaum and Dr. Cary Goldberg and known as The Center for Dental Excellence. My family and I have been patients of this dental group for over 20 years. Their expertise, personal attention and state-of-the-art equipment provide optimum care. As a busy attorney, I appreciate their staff who are courteous, friendly, professional and most accommodating in booking appointments. I highly recommend

CDE to my clients, friends and family. I am positive patients will receive the most advanced, pain-free treatments to solve their dental problems. As I have.

Arnold Newman
Of Counsel Attorney at Law
Newman, Boyer & Statham, Ltd.
Greater Chicago Area

I have known Doctors Goldberg and Greenebaum professionally and personally for over 20 years and can truly say that they just keep getting better. Their exceptional skills combined with a top-notch staff deliver quality dental solutions that exceed expectations. If you are looking for a beautiful smile, then their office is a must!

Dr. John Saniat, Owner
Practice Limited to Periodontics
Wheaton, Illinois

I highly recommend Dr. Goldberg and Dr. Greenbaum. I have been practicing in the dental industry for over 35 years and have worked with over 300 doctors. I know what to look for in a dental practice and these two have got it. They are both highly skilled, learning the latest techniques with numerous hours of continuing education. Their equipment, facility and staff are second to none. If you wanted to find a dental home with passion, compassion, trust and a place where you can be treated fairly, look no further.

Mike Capps, CDT, President
Technic Dental Lab, Inc.
Orland Park, IL

The Flossmoor area's foremost dental practice in complete implant restoration, as well as Hollywood-Smile cosmetic makeovers is The Center for Dental Excellence. Owned by Dr.

Cary Goldberg and Dr. Charles Greenebaum, their extensive knowledge and precision in helping to solve complex dental problems through restorative implants and cosmetic dentistry puts them at the top of their field and truly sets them apart from the rest. They continue to transform the lives of thousands of patients, providing world-class care. The doctors and their team create an atmosphere of warmth and exceptional hospitality where all are treated like family from the moment they enter the doors. Doctors Goldberg and Greenebaum are two of the most positive and caring individuals you will ever meet. It is no wonder that patients travel from around the country to seek out their services. Going to the dentist never felt so good!

Dr. Lisa Grant, Owner
Lisa Grant Orthodontics
Homewood, Illinois

I have been fortunate to have worked with Dr. Goldberg and Dr. Greenebaum and the doctors at CDE for many years now and can say without reservation that they provide the highest quality of care for their patients. As a specialist who works with many dentists in the area, I find the doctors at CDE to be talented professionals with excellent clinical skills and expertise. I am always comfortable that when one of their patients comes into my office, the patient has had a complete, thorough, comprehensive evaluation with treatment planning that has the patient's best interest at heart. The doctors at CDE take pride in not cutting corners and providing the best dentistry possible in a caring environment.

George E. Morris, Jr., D.D.S
Oral & Maxillofacial Surgery
Homewood, Illinois

The Center for Dental Excellence exemplifies the State of the Art in dentistry. It resonates the highest quality of dental care that is second to none. Dr. Goldberg, Dr. Greenebaum & Associates collectively provide customized dental care for each patient individually with compassion, trust, and the goal to make every patient's experience a grateful one. Their vast experience and expertise in cosmetic, implant and general dentistry affords their patients a unique opportunity to be the recipients of special care. The outstanding dental team, which includes those at the front desk and telephone, dental assistants, and those behind the scenes, are truly professional and generate a warm and caring atmosphere to instill each patient with a pleasant and comfortable experience. This practice is the finest dental office that I have been affiliated with in my forty years of private practice.

Robert D. Schwartz, B.S. D.M.D., F.A.C.D.

www.ingramcontent.com/pod-product-compliance
Lightning Source LLC
Chambersburg PA
CBHW071039240526
45469CB00006BD/2272